Treating Teenage Drug Abuse in a Day Care Setting

Treating Teenage Drug Abuse in a Day Care Setting

William Feigelman

Foreword by David E. Smith

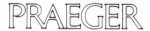

New York
Westport, Connecticut
London

Library of Congress Cataloging-in-Publication Data

Feigelman, William.
    Treating teenage drug abuse in a day care setting / William Feigelman.
        p.   cm.
    Includes bibliographical references.
    ISBN 0-275-93379-2 (alk. paper)
    1. Teenagers—New York (State)—Nassau County—Drug use—Case
studies. 2. Narcotic addicts—Rehabilitation—New York (State)—
Manhasset—Case studies. 3. Drug abuse—Treatment—New York
(State)—Manhasset—Case studies. I. Title.
    HV5824.Y68F43   1990
    362.29'185'09747245—dc20   89-26538

Library of Congress Catalog Card Number: 89-26538
ISBN: 0-275-93379-2

First published in 1990

Praeger Publishers, One Madison Avenue, New York, NY 10010
A division of Greenwood Press, Inc.

Printed in the United States of America

The paper used in this book complies with the Permanent
Paper Standard issued by the National Information Standards
Organization (Z39.48–1984).

10   9   8   7   6   5   4   3   2   1

*For Beverly, whose continual love
and caring lights my way.*

Contents

Tables

Foreword

Treating Teenage Drug Abuse in a Day Care Setting deals with some of the most complicated contemporary issues in addiction treatment.

Day treatment is a treatment modality of growing importance in completing the continuum of care, but it has not been described with the depth seen in this book. The problem of adolescent drug abuse has been aptly documented, but treatment outcome particularly treatment outcome of adolescent addiction has not been adequately studied.

This monograph provides an excellent conceptual framework for understanding the basis of day treatment for teenagers. A strong methodology chapter provides the basis for evaluating its effectiveness. Outcome variables are described in depth thus serving as the basis for analyzing treatment outcome results.

In the addiction treatment field we need to expand new treatment approaches such as day treatment and we need to better understand what correlates with effective adolescent treatment. Dr. Feigelman's rigorous scientific approach outline in his monograph advances knowledge in both areas. I hope that such knowledge will serve as the basis of effective treatment for drug abusing adolescents.

David E. Smith, President and Medical Director
Haight Ashbury Free Clinics, Inc.
San Francisco, California

Acknowledgments

During the long course of work on this project I received much valuable aid. I would like to take this opportunity to thank the many people who helped with their very substantial acts of assistance. Indeed, without these many contributions of time, talent, and support, this book would never have been possible.

First, I would like to thank Ken Amann of Long Island Jewish Medical Center and Steve Rutter of Queens General Hospital. They initially inspired me to embark upon this study, encouraged me to think that it could be done and then later conducted some of the follow-up interviews with former day care patients. Ken was especially helpful in securing permission to do the research with the administration of Long Island Jewish-Hillside Medical Center and their Human Subjects Review Committee. I am especially grateful to the leadership of the Medical Center for their cooperation and encouragement. When an outsider such as myself enters the inner ranks of an organization in order to study one of its programs, there is always some element of wariness that its objectives may be misunderstood or unduly criticized. Yet, in this particular case, the only concerns expressed by hospital administration were that the research findings would ultimately improve the quality of patient care.

I am particularly grateful to the Sabbatical Leave Committee at Nassau Community College for the leave I was awarded in 1986; their grant greatly accelerated my pace in completing this work.

This book evolved from my doctoral dissertation research which was done in the Sociology Department at the State University of New York at Stony Brook. I am especially grateful to the faculty members who served on my doctoral committee: Paul Attewell, Erich Goode, and Kenneth Feldman. I was very fortunate to have such an extremely capable and generous group of advisors. Throughout the study's long course, Paul Attewell never flagged in his availability, interest, and support. His aid was especially important in formulating the experimental design and in improving preliminary and final drafts of the analysis. His encouragement was constant and his critical suggestions always intelligent, painstaking, and valuable. Erich Goode, also, was especially generous with his time. He helped me take a more systematic and global perspective of the findings. When my text began to read too much like "dis-

sertationese," he gently guided me toward the creation of a more literate for-
mulation.

Merton Hyman, an associate at the Center for Alcohol Studies at Rutgers
University and longtime friend, was a godsend. He was always ready to read
my many drafts, never hesitated to perform statistical recalculations, and con-
stantly offered careful and considered criticism of the study throughout its
many phases. Hyman was especially helpful in guiding me to become more
knowledgeable and proficient with the statistical aspects of the research and
with using SPSS. Bernard Gorman, one of my Nassau College colleagues, also
helped me thread my way through the statistical maze.

I am also deeply in debt to the several people who served as research assist-
ants on the project; they completed a good many of the follow-up interviews.
Although a few received nominal payments for their services, an obvious love
of learning and a desire to help inspired them to make their very generous contributions of time and effort. Sarah Keyes, Marion Mallah, Edythe Scro, and
Catherine Ward all gave very generously of themselves. Judy Ouellette, a counselor at the Manhasset Community Day Center, was very helpful on many occasions, filling me in on important historical details about the program and
assisting in finding files of terminated patients.

My wife Beverly was another very important source of aid. She never tired
of reading and rereading my countless drafts and always found ways to improve the quality of the writing. Her extensive experience as a drug rehabilitation therapist enabled me to make sense of the sometimes bewildering information I accumulated from counselors at the Manhasset Community Day
Center and their former patients. I am amazed that she still tolerates me after
all my endless questions, musings, and downright obsessiveness.

Last, but by no means least, I would like to express my gratitude to the many
former patient respondents who gave so freely of their time and shared with
the research staff so many intimate details of their personal lives. Without
their cooperation, a study would not have been possible. Although the interviews took much time to administer, most respondents remained available to
provide additional important anecdotal information. Their great cooperation
helped immeasurably.

Treating Teenage Drug Abuse in a Day Care Setting

1

Introduction

Day Care Treatment for Adolescent Drug Abusers: A Neglected Area of Inquiry

Ever since the late 1950s adolescent substance abuse has emerged as a national problem of immense proportions. Social researchers have amply documented the growing incidence of polydrug abuse among teenagers (Radosevich, Lanza-Kaduce, Akers, and Krohn, 1979). Yet the ways adolescents may be effectively treated for their substance-abusing behavior remain less well known (Beschner and Friedman, 1985). Outpatient programs, one of the commonly used treatment approaches, are probably one of the least well understood modes for promoting rehabilitation.

There is a considerable and growing body of literature on clients who have been patients in drug treatment programs. A great deal is now known about the modalities of methadone maintenance and therapeutic communities. Evidence is also beginning to accumulate on the longer-term outcomes of drug treatment (Collier and Hijazi, 1974; Pin, Martin, and Walsh, 1976; DeLeon, 1984; Dole and Joseph, 1978; Maddux and McDonald, 1973); Stimmel et al., 1978; Bale et al., 1980; Burt Associates, Inc., 1977; Vaillant, 1978; Simpson and Sells, 1982; Simpson et al., 1986; Hubbard et al., 1984; Rush, 1979).

Study results clearly show that whatever the particular mode—whether methadone maintenance, therapeutic community, or outpatient drug-free programs—treatment usually succeeds (Tims, 1981). For most of the studies treatment successes are measured in terms of three elements: reduction in the use of drugs, reduced criminality, and increased productive activity, such as job holding or attending school.

To give the reader some idea of the magnitude of the successes, Collier and Hijazi (1974) did a follow-up of patients treated for approximately twenty months at Daytop Village, a residential facility in New York, which took place about a year after treatment. They found that among those opiate-abusing patients completing treatment 84% were not using drugs, had not been arrested, and were employed or going to school a year later. The remaining 16% also showed some signs of improvement over their earlier pretreatment state.

Among program dropouts, however, only 46% were drug- and crime-free and employed or in school a year later. Pin, Martin, and Walsh (1976) evaluated a therapeutic community and day care program for heroin addicts in New York City. They concluded:

"Success" is related to the length of time the ex-client spent in the treatment program: among the ex-clients who stayed in treatment three months or less, 54.7% were found jobless, 74.5% were back on [hard] drugs, and 57.2% had been arrested; on the other hand, among those who remained in treatment for more than a year, only 6.8% were jobless, 3.9% had returned to drugs, and 23.2% had been arrested. (p. 403)

Such indications of treatment success have usually been obtained comparing treated respondents with matched controls that did not remain in treatment (Collier and Hijazi, 1974; Pin, Martin, and Walsh, 1976; DeLeon, 1984; Dole and Joseph, 1978; Maddux and McDonald, 1973; Stimmel et al., 1978; Bale et al., 1980). These and other studies have found treated patients doing significantly better—in terms of study criteria—than those dropping out. Most of these positive results have been obtained in shorter term follow-ups done about a year after program termination.

Yet, it should be noted that most programs encounter considerable attrition among their initial entering patients (Tims, 1981). It is not unusual to find anywhere from a third to half of entering patients withdrawing from treatment within the first few months of care. According to DeLeon and Schwartz (1984), among the 1979 admissions to all federally-funded treatment programs, twelve-month retention rates averaged 22% in methadone maintenance, 9% in drug-free ambulatory programs, and 7% in drug-free residential programs.

Given such pervasive treatment departures one might conclude that much of contemporary drug care is ineffective in inspiring the participation of the largest numbers of those plagued by substance abuse problems. By this criteria most contemporary treatments could be viewed as failures. Their successes are confined to a minority of highly motivated entrants. Yet for these populations, success appears to be well established (Tims, 1981).

Methadone maintenance, therapeutic communities, and outpatient drug-free modalities appear to achieve more dramatic treatment results than detoxification. Given its less intensive nature and usually shorter duration, detoxification has been singularly less effective. One follow-up study of detoxification (Simpson, Savage, and Sells, 1978) consisting of up to twenty-one days of care noted that over half (54%) returned to daily opioid use during the first year after detoxification; and 68% returned to some opioid use. Thus, longer courses of treatment are more likely to be successful than shorter ones (DeLeon, 1984; Sells and Simpson, 1979).

Surveying the available studies on adolescent drug rehabilitation it is apparent that there is a dearth of information on drug-free outpatient and day care treatments (Tims, 1981; Beschner and Friedman, 1985). It also remains uncertain which types of clients, from which kinds of family and social backgrounds, benefit most from these approaches. Even less well known are the longer-term results of this form of care. The present research attempts to address all of these issues.

There appears to be no published literature available on day care treatment for polydrug-abusing adolescents. There are several studies available indicating day care's utility in treating adult alcoholics and narcotic addicts (McLachlan and Stein, 1982; Fox and Lowe, 1968; Collins, Watson, and Zrimec, 1980; Bensinger and Pilkington, 1983; Kaufman, 1972; Kissin and Sang, 1973; Kleber, 1970). Available studies suggest that day care is an effective and cost-saving alternative to residential treatment or hospitalization. For example, McLachlan and Stein (1982) studied one hundred Canadian alcoholics completing day treatment and inpatient care and found that a total of 58% had stopped drinking at follow-up. Half the patients had been randomly assigned to day care and the remainder received inpatient treatment. Among all patients 33% were completely abstinent for a year, and 25% had brief relapses of no more than a total of fourteen total drinking days from which they recovered. Another 28% had significantly reduced their intake (compared to pre-intake consumption levels), and 11% had relapsed completely. They found that the numbers of improved day care patients were very similar to the numbers improving from inpatient care as well as statistically undifferentiated. However, the day care program was much more cost-effective; it was 65% less costly to operate per patient than the inpatient program.

However, no studies have been done to describe and evaluate the day care approach in treating teenage multidrug abuse. No doubt the paucity of a day care literature reflects the general pattern that most teenagers receiving drug care are either enrolled in residential or conventional outpatient treatments. Beschner and Friedman (1985) report that relatively few of the 51,000-plus teenagers undergoing drug treatments now receive day care. George Beschner (1986) claims that there are only about fifty such day care programs available nationally, compared to the hundreds or more residential programs and thousands of outpatient treatment facilities. Clearly, day care represents a less utilized treatment modality. With a fuller understanding of this approach, and its beneficiaries, there may be justification for expanding its availability. Demonstrations of its utility in adolescent care could possibly bring similar cost-saving advantages over residential treatments found in treating other substance abuse problems.

Day Care: A Middle Ground of Drug Therapy

Day care is an uncommon form of treatment for teenage drug abuse. It is less intensive and encompassing in the control it exerts over patients than is possible in a residential treatment facility. In residential therapeutic communities young drug abusers can be completely isolated from their drug-using peer groups. The treatment center can also readily regulate the amount of association between adolescent patients and their families.

When parents promote drug abuse by offering youngsters deviant role models, or by their own normative dissension and confusion, patients can be removed from such abuse-inspiring settings. Residential treatment facilities try to change the patient's behavior by any number of therapeutic approaches: conventional psychotherapies, peer confrontation, behavior conditioning, academic and vocational counseling, drug education programs, and milieu therapies, among other treatments. If the residential program is within traveling distance of the patient's family, then they, too, can be direct participants in the therapeutic process.

The residential approach can induce behavioral change among its clients by the various therapies it applies and the nearly total control it exerts over the individual patient. One of the problems that has been recognized in applying this modality is in reconciling the fundamental dissimilarities between the heavily controlled atmosphere of the treatment center and the less structured larger society. Many patients ultimately encounter difficulty in trying to readjust in the society outside the treatment facility. Of course, administrators of therapeutic communities recognize this issue and address it by creating any number of transitional stages of "reentry" status to prepare the individual for conventional social participation. Yet, despite such interim stages many clients still encounter difficulties in changing from successfully adapted clients into drug-free civilians.

At the other end of the spectrum there are conventional outpatient therapies, where the client is permitted to function in their home environment and to regularly attend the treatment facility for psychotherapy, counseling, or advisement. In most outpatient programs for teenage drug abuse parents are also expected to be co-participants in the treatment process. Family therapy is usually provided, in addition to the diverse individual treatments given. Usually, outpatient therapies are available to clients whose level of abuse is less acutely problematic, and who are not considered to be as dangerous to society or to themselves; thus, they may benefit from less control of their conduct, and a greater opportunity to work out their difficulties within the civilian society. In outpatient treatment, efforts are directed toward working with clients in their home environments as they attempt to realize their drug-free (or drug-reduced) goals.

In contrast to both of these approaches day care can be seen as the middle ground of treatment. In day care, patients are supervised at the treatment facility during the work day, then return to their homes during evening and weekend hours. This treatment mode is a more controlling and intrusive intervention than is possible in a series of regular visits to a therapist/counselor/ therapy group, as in outpatient care. By dealing with its clients who form a somewhat remote part of the civilian society when they are in treatment, the day care center may avoid some of the adjustment difficulties that trouble patients upon release from residential programs. The day care center must rely heavily upon parental resources to monitor the progress of treatment and to provide for the realization of treatment objectives when clients are not at the treatment facility.

It remains uncertain how effective this approach is in treating teenage poly-drug abuse. Many questions arise in relation to the appropriate administration of a day care program. What must be expected in parental participation? How closely must parents monitor their child in order to achieve treatment objectives? What must program administrators do to inspire the necessary levels of parental cooperation and commitment that will promote treatment success? How closely must other family members be supervised by the treatment center to facilitate treatment success? Must parents and other siblings be drug-free if the treatment goals are to be achieved? And which patients and families are most likely to gain from this treatment modality which emphasizes family involvements? Conversely, which groups and persons are not likely to be helped by this treatment approach, who would be best served by programs dealing more directly with patients, and independently of their particular familial resources? These additional questions invite further exploration.

Every year more than 51,000 adolescents begin treatment for substance abuse problems (Beschner and Friedman, 1985). All will be treated in a variety of residential, day care, and outpatient programs. Yet little is known about how the different kinds of programs work, how they manage to help their clientele, and which clients benefit most from the different programs that are available. And even less is known about the effectiveness of these treatments over the long term. If day care can be shown to be an effective type of treatment, greater use may be made of it in the future. With greater knowledge of those who are likely to benefit from this form of treatment, better treatment placement decisions can be made.

Almost all available studies on outpatient adolescent drug treatment were conducted within a year after treatment was concluded (Rush, 1979; Hubbard et al., 1983; Mai et al., 1980; Winn, 1981). Only one study followed patients up to four to six years after admission (Sells and Simpson, 1979). It is imperative that more longer treatment evaluations be conducted if we are to fully understand the value of these treatments.

Post-treatment Behavior: Variations in Adjustments and the Role of Drug Use in Post-treatment Adaptations

The existing body of research evidence suggests that while most who undergo outpatient drug-free treatment are likely to improve in their social functioning, most resume drug-taking. Usually, the drug-taking subsequent to treatment involves "soft" drug use, such as marijuana and alcohol. And even these drugs may be used in smaller quantities than before treatment (Sells and Simpson, 1979; Hubbard et al., 1983). In the Drug Abuse Reporting Program (DARP) study (Sells and Simpson, 1979) it was noted that between 20% and 46% of subsamples reduced their use of opiates after treatment. Arrests also dropped to between 40% and 45%. Yet alcohol and marijuana use remained undiminished after treatment for whites, and increased slightly for black respondents. The Treatment Outcome Prospective Study (TOPS) (Hubbard et al., 1983) found that more than one-third reported not using their pretreatment primary drug during the follow-up period. Involvements in criminal activities also diminished from 53% to 36% of respondents, yet the research also found more daily marijuana users at follow-up (54%) than in the year preceding treatment (48%). Heavy alcohol use declined, but not dramatically, with 54% at intake and 41% at follow-up.

Questions arise from these findings about the significance of post-treatment drug use. If frequent marijuana and alcohol use still occurs among those completing treatments, can we still regard such patients as recovered? Is this an indication that treatment is falling short of expectations? Or, is it possible that some post-treatment drug experimentation and use is inevitable but not necessarily a sign of treatment failure? Examining the linkages between post-treatment drug use and other aspects of individual functioning should be very helpful in assessing the quality of recoveries. How are the differences in patterns of post-treatment drug use correlated with other aspects of individual behavior: criminality, educational attainments, work behavior, mental and physical health status, and overall social integration? What are the distinctive characteristics of those who return to drug use but who are able to function in an otherwise acceptable way in the community? How are they differentiated from others, who also revert to drug-taking, but who are out of control and functioning less well? And what about those former patients who permanently abstain from psychoactive drug use altogether? What are their distinctive social characteristics? How can each of these three groups be more readily identified? These questions are explored in the pages that follow.

Day Care Patients: A Basis for Exploring Other Questions about Adolescent Substance Abuse

Studying a population of patients admitted for day care presents a rich opportunity for exploring a broad array of questions about the nature and causes of substance abuse, as well as treatments for it. Many pretreatment characteristics of clients and their families have been linked with initial treatment outcomes. Ages at first drinking and getting drunk, performance in school prior to onset of drug problems, history of delinquent involvements, depression at entry, and other individual-based characteristics have been established in previous research as correlates of youth drug abuse (Brunswick and Boyle, 1979; Kleinman, 1978; Johnston et al., 1978; Kandel et al., 1976; Jessor and Jessor, 1977). One may also wonder whether such factors exert an influence upon the persistence of drug abuse. Do such factors continue to have a bearing on drug abuse after former patients have reached their middle twenties, years after completing drug treatments?

It is almost axiomatic in the drug rehabilitation field that unless patients are motivated to obtain treatment, drug therapy is not likely to be successful. Several studies have found that the greater the number of attempts patients make to get help and the longer they remain in care, the greater their chances of giving up drugs (Pin, Martin, and Walsh, 1976; Simpson, 1979). Furthermore, voluntary patients are more likely to succeed in treatment than those referred by the courts (Stimmel et al., 1978). Stimmel et al. found 22% of their voluntarily detoxified subjects narcotic-free at follow-up, compared to only 5% of those detoxified because of arrest. However, most of this research has been conducted among older drug abusers and those receiving treatment for opioid abuse. It remains to be demonstrated whether motivational commitments play a similar role in the drug abuse and rehabilitation of youthful polydrug abusers. This research investigates whether the motivations for getting treatment are linked with completing day care and long-term recovery from youth drug abuse.

Coping with the experience of parental divorce, parent-child conflict during adolescence, and parental inconsistency have been found in other studies to be important contributors to explaining patterns of substance abuse (Jessor and Jessor, 1977; Brook, Lukoff, and Whiteman, 1980; Kandel, Kessler and Margulies, 1978; Robins, Davis, and Wish, 1977). Examining the importance of these factors both for completing the day care treatment modality and in longer-term drug rehabilitations provides valuable information.

Previous research has provided ample documentation that parental misuse of drugs is an important correlate of adolescent substance abuse (Brook et al., 1977, 1978; Kandel et al., 1978). Yet it remains to be demonstrated whether parental abstinence can be employed therapeutically in controlling adolescent substance abuse. One of the goals of this study will be to investigate whether families varying in their abstinence during their child's treatment are likely to contribute to differing results in post-treatment outcomes.

Administrators of many day care and outpatient programs generally agree that drug therapy without familial support would not be very effective. These assumptions about the importance of the family in drug rehabilitation have been supported in a number of clinical studies (Reilly, 1975; Huberty, 1975; Noone and Reddig, 1976; Stanton et al., 1978; Hendin, Pollinger, Ulman, and Carr, 1981). Nevertheless, many aspects of parental behavior and involvement in their children's treatment remain empirically unexamined. How important are family participation, involvement, and cooperation with treatment for promoting treatment objectives? Are they indispensable for effective treatment, as many drug program administrators would claim? Could favorable outcomes result without parental participation, commitment, and cooperation? Can the single parent, or the parent in a reconstituted marriage, accomplish as much toward furthering the day treatment objectives of their child as parents of intact marriages? These questions are empirically examined in this study.

Thus, this exploratory analysis will attempt to add new knowledge about the adolescent populations likely to seek, complete, and benefit from day care drug therapy. Hopefully, the information will prove useful for promoting a more efficient allocation of professional and familial resources to ultimately provide more effective adolescent drug treatments.

The Research Setting and the Population Studied: The Manhasset Community Day Center

The Manhasset Community Day Center presents an interesting site for studying the problems of drug abuse and rehabilitation. The program—one of several substance abuse treatment facilities offered by Long Island Jewish-Hillside Medical Center—provides care for adolescent substance abusers and their families in Nassau County, New York. It is geared to serving polydrug abusers between the ages of twelve and nineteen. The treatment center is located in the Christ Episcopal Church on Northern Boulevard in Manhasset.

The Manhasset Community Day Center has some distinctive features. For one, it services one of the richest counties in the nation. It draws its clientele from the affluent populations of Long Island's North Shore and from the predominantly middle class communities of Nassau County. Although there are several poverty pockets within the region, poorer families form a decidedly smaller segment of the community and the treatment population.

The MCDC program offers two different treatment modes: day treatment or outpatient care. Day care is usually reserved for those adolescents with the following characteristics: younger persons of high school age, those presenting relatively serious drug abuse problems, situations where family members show great commitment to treatment, and those with a previous history of treatment for drug abuse.

The focus of the study was on the day care treatment mode. In the absence of any available literature on day care treatment for teenage drug abuse, how typical the Manhasset program may be among the variety of other day care treatments offered nationally is unclear. This description may be a useful point of departure in any future discussions of this subject.

The Manhasset Community Day Center program began treating adolescents in 1974. Although it is administered by Long Island Jewish-Hillside Medical Center, funding is provided by Nassau County. Patients' families are also charged fees for treatment on a sliding scale depending upon family incomes. The maximum fee for a family for treatment is ninety-five dollars per week. Indigent families can receive completely subsidized care.

At any given time, the center usually contains a population of up to 40 adolescents in day care and a somewhat smaller number in treatment as outpatients. Since it started, more than eight hundred adolescents and their families have been associated with the program; about half (four hundred) were initially accepted for day care. The total day care population actually exceeded this number; some patients, initially accepted for outpatient treatment, eventually entered day care.

For this research a complete list was created of all patients entering treatment by 1984 who had ever been enrolled in the day care program. It was noted that not all treatment files covering the early years of the center's operation were still available. However, treatment files spanning back to 1977 were still available in their entirety. This became the beginning cut point and 1984 was established as the terminus. A four-digit identification number was assigned to each patient's family. Then, with a table of random numbers a two-thirds sample was selected from this entire population, yielding a total sample of 184 cases. Thus, during this time period a total of 276 patients were accepted into day care.

Typically, adolescent patients enter the day care program as polydrug abusers, with the greatest numbers abusing marijuana, alcohol, hallucinogens, barbiturates, amphetamines, and cocaine. Sampled patients listed these drugs, in descending order, as among the three they most frequently used when they entered treatment. Table 1-1 lists the three chiefly abused drugs of Manhasset day care patients and the percentage having ever used each type of drug. (Since 1984, prevailing drug abuse patterns at the treatment center have kept pace with national changes in youth drug abuse. Nowadays, cocaine has become the third most commonly listed drug among post-1984 day care patients.) The sample of patients drawn from clinic files showed the following patterns of drug abuse at intake: three fourths of sampled patients took their chiefly abused drug at least daily; an additional 14% used drugs at least several times a week. The extensiveness of drug-taking among those entering treatment was also reflected in the pattern of 43% found to be taking their mainly abused drug at least two to three times daily.

At the time of entry into the program, parents usually recognized that their child was "out of control." Children may have been stealing possessions belonging to their parents, engaging in persistent truancy, or having some other trouble with the courts or juvenile authorities. Crimes were not unusual among this clinic population: over half (52%) had committed serious criminal offenses, such as burglary, assault, theft, gun possession, in addition to drug-related offenses. Most (71%) had a prior arrest experience, although most arrestees committed a variety of drug and juvenile status offenses.

Among the sample it was noted that nearly half (49%) were placed in the program's custody in response to a court or probation order, as an alternative to more confined treatment or incarceration. Included within this group were some who were required to participate by PINS petitions. A PINS petition is

Table 1-1.
Drug Use at Intake

Type of Drug	Percent using drug
marijuana	93
alcohol	48
hallucinogens	34
barbiturates	31
amphetamines	25
cocaine	16
sedatives	9
PCP	7
tranquilizers	4
inhalants	2
heroin	2
methadone	0
other opiates	0
over-the-counter drugs	0

a court order issued usually by a local juvenile court attesting to the delinquent conduct of a youth; PINS stands for a 'person in need of supervision.' An additional 41% were referred to the program by a school, hospital, or other social agency. In many of these latter instances, if families remained opposed to program involvement, the particular agency might have applied for a court order to mandate participation. Either the child's parents or the home school, or local law enforcement agencies who recognized the child's unmanageability, insisted that the child participate in the program. Only about 10% of sampled clients were voluntary admissions.

Complete abstinence from nonprescribed drugs is demanded from all of those in day care treatment. Since the program's inception, the prevailing treatment philosophy has been one favoring abstinence. The belief has been, and remains, that there is no safe or acceptable level of drug use for teenagers while under treatment. When day care treatment is concluded, moderate use of alcohol is seen as acceptable for adult former patients, unless counter-indicated because of alcoholism.

Upon entry into treatment close adherence to program rules is anticipated. Any deviations from treatment rules, especially those committed by program newcomers, are taken as serious infractions. Behavior involving drug use, the program's central focus, is a possible ground for termination. At any time, staff members may require clients to provide a urine specimen (under supervision) to verify their drug-free condition.

To achieve its goal of drug-free living, the program employs a variety of treatment approaches. It offers group and individual therapy, peer confrontation, family counseling, behavioral conditioning, physical activities, insight training, vocational guidance, and drug reeducation. Manhasset Community Day Center also coordinates the provision of on-site high school classes so that youngsters can complete their high school programs while they receive treatment.

Another distinctive component of treatment at Manhasset Community Day Center is the heavy demand placed upon parents as participants in their child's rehabilitation. The patients' parents and siblings are expected to abstain altogether from drug use during treatment, and are also not permitted to consume alcoholic beverages during the early phases of therapy. At no time during the course of the child's treatment, of up to three years, are alcoholic beverages permitted in the home.

The monitoring of parental and sibling abstinence is a difficult task. Yet, within the intimate environment of the family many lapses in drug use are brought to the attention of other family members. These violations are likely to be discussed in one of the ongoing treatment experiences and contacts: individual counseling sessions, parent meetings, and group therapy. Once suspicions are raised about a particular parent's drug abstinence they, too, are asked to provide urine specimens for chemical identification of drug residues. Urines are then collected from them on an intermittent basis, until their willingness to conform to program expectations is demonstrated. Parents violating program abstinence rules are normally sanctioned. For initial offenses, they are usually asked to attend several additional parental rules sessions or denied carpooling privileges. If drug use persists, then program termination of the family becomes the inevitable result. However, termination can be averted when other drug-using family members agree to participate in some additional outpatient treatment to address their drug or alcohol problems.

Every weekend, on a rotating basis, parents are entrusted with the care of their child and two or three other children in the program. It is assumed that a child with a history of drug abuse must be monitored continually, lest he/she resume contact with former drug-abusing peers and revert to drug use. Children are not even permitted to take the family dog for a walk unless accompanied by a responsible adult. When their children are not under the program's supervision, parents are obliged to know their child's whereabouts at all times. Other therapeutic demands placed upon parents include weekly participation in group therapy which continues for the duration of their child's treatment.

Families must possess a modicum of economic resources to participate in the treatment regimen. They must have access to an automobile to provide transportation to and from the program. They must be able to accommodate three to four teenagers in their domicile for the weekend on a rotating basis. They must be able to get along financially without the income of their teenager who is undergoing treatment, since teenagers in day treatment are prohibited from having jobs. Any activity that cannot be closely supervised, such as outside work, is not permitted. Parents unable to comply with these program requirements would be referred to an alternative treatment facility.

In day care programs patients spend most of their time at the treatment facility, but return to sleep at home. Children remain at the center from 8:30 A.M. till 5:00 P.M. At the center they engage in a round of activities consisting of regular classroom sessions (mathematics, science, English, social studies, typing, health, etc.) and recreation (athletics and physical exercise).

Each child has a set of assigned activities in the running of the program, such as sweeping the hallways, making coffee, serving as telephone receptionist, painting offices, or working in the garden. As the child shows progress in treatment he or she is given greater trust, responsibility, and status. As progress is demonstrated, a teenager is given an opportunity to offer guidance and direction to new patients, to represent the treatment facility to the outside community, or another such assignment, reflecting the level of accomplishment he/she has attained in treatment. The child's involvement in a variety of therapeutic experiences—group therapy, individual counseling, family counseling, behavior modification training, and drug reeducation classes—is integrated with work activities.

Usually day care treatment lasts from fourteen to eighteen months. When adolescents and their families are judged to have completed the course of treatment, youngsters move into a new status known as "reentry." During the reentry phase, adolescents function more independently in the community. They may return to their neighborhood schools or hold outside employment, while continuing group therapy and drug reeducation courses at the center. During the time period of the study, when patients were in reentry, those of legal age could also request social drinking privileges.

The program population was predominately male (68%) during the course of the study period. Ninety-three percent of entering patients were white, non-Hispanics. Nearly two-fifths of fathers worked at professional, managerial, or entrepreneurial occupations. An additional two-fifths were employed as white-collar or skilled manual workers. Fifty-seven percent of families were Catholic, 14% Protestant, and 26% Jewish. Aside from the overrepresentation of males in the program, the treatment population is not greatly dissimilar from the overall demographics of Nassau County.[1]

Given the heavy demands placed upon participating families and individuals it should be no surprise to learn that the majority of clients do not complete the course of treatment. Only 14% of the sample completed treatment and were "graduated" from the program. This figure is slightly higher than what has been reported for the completion rate in (adolescent and adult) therapeutic community programs, which is said to be about 9% to 10% (DeLeon, 1984). Among those completing the course of day care treatment, clients' range of time in the program varied from a low of nineteen months to a high of thirty-nine. Of all clients initially assigned to day care, 52% withdrew from treatment within the first six months; an additional 14% received care for more than six months but less than a year; 22% were given treatment from between one and two years; and 12% stayed in treatment for longer than two years.

Experiencing Day Care: Some Case Illustrations

As one enters the Manhasset Day Center one encounters an unusual place. It is a combination school, camp, prison, mental health clinic, social club, and amusement center all rolled into one. Having described the workings of the Manhasset Day Center, let us now look at a few illustrative cases that show how patients personally experience day care. In all case illustrations names and significant personal details have been changed to protect the privacy rights of the actual persons mentioned.

Case No. 1: Carla Greenspan

Carla entered the Manhasset program about a year-and-a-half ago at age thirteen. When she was admitted she smoked marijuana several times weekly and drank alcohol heavily. At that time, she was on the verge of being suspended from junior high school because of truancy and poor academic performance. On most school days Carla would party with friends, spend her time at a friend's empty house, drink beer, smoke joints, and listen to music. During such occasions, as opportunities presented themselves, Carla also had sex with an assortment of male partners.

Being aware of and deeply concerned about her school problems, Carla's parents drove her to school every day on their way to work. However, their efforts were futile, because, after she was dropped off, Carla generally left school. Her parents were dimly aware of Carla's history of sexual acting out and her heavy drug-taking. In the past her parents had taken Carla for private psychotherapy on two occasions. Each time, however, these efforts failed to get her involved in therapy.

Mr. and Mrs. Greenspan were both professionals and high achievers: her father, a successful accountant; her mother, a high school principal. Both parents held especially high academic expectations for their daughter. Her older brother was an honors student, and they expected similar accomplishments from Carla. When it finally became clear just how grave Carla's school problems were both parents and Carla unloaded on each other. Carla defiantly let her parents know about her drug use and sexual exploits. Her parents threatened to have her sent to a home for wayward youth or to an ultrastrict boarding school. Carla threatened to leave home and go out on her own. When tempers cooled, and after some checking around about community resources, it was eventually decided that MCDC would be the best place for

Carla. She could be helped to give up drugs and get back on an academic track, and the family could work toward resolving its differences.

Carla's initial feelings about going to the day center were mixed. On the one hand, she liked and admired some of the counselors and patients that she met during her first few visits. On the other hand, she hated all the rules and restrictions which kept her from doing her own thing. She acknowledged her deep confusion, but felt that the center presented a better alternative than leaving home and going to some distant and unfamiliar boarding school.

Since Carla's admission into the day center she has been neither a model patient, nor a special problem case. Shortly after she began treatment she ran away from the center for a few hours with another male patient. When she returned she accepted her disciplinary consequences: isolation from her peers when not in class or therapy. After that incident and during the next several months she demonstrated treatment progress, did well in school, showed no evidence of any drug use, and generally displayed positive attitudes to staff and other patients. As her behavior improved, she was given additional privileges and freedoms.

After approximately a year of steady progress a minor incident developed when she criticized a staff member disrespectfully. For this infraction she was told to remain seated on a prospect chair (social isolation) for the remainder of the afternoon. At the other end of the room another patient, a male, was sitting out his time on another prospect chair for his own infraction. Carla tried to induce this peer to leave the center with her. When he refused, Carla, without provocation, attacked him. Nearby patients eventually intervened and stopped the attack with the assistance of staff. This physically aggressive outburst represented a serious breach of program discipline, for which Carla was immediately suspended and her parents notified.

Later a special staff meeting was held to discuss Carla's behavior and decide whether she should be referred out of the program. While some staff members favored such a course of action it was eventually decided—considering her past progress and the highly cooperative response of her parents—to give Carla another chance. Standing before a general meeting of her peers Carla was told that she had lost all her previously earned privileges and would be on cleanup detail for the next month. Also, she would have to cover her hair with a nylon stocking cap. (The use of the stocking cap is derived from the therapeutic community intervention of shaving someone's hair after the violation of a serious program rule. In the day treatment center a stocking cap has been substituted for the shaved head. The concept behind the intervention: one must pay something [one's hair] to be accepted back into the program family.)

So far Carla seems to have accepted her punishment. Her counselor has told her that if she continues to function well she will soon be able to reclaim her former relatively privileged patient status. He has also assured her that there is the possibility she may still be able to apply for reentry status within three to four months. It remains uncertain what Carla's eventual fate with day care treatment will be; it is obvious that Carla must still work on several behavioral issues.

Recent interviews with her indicate that Carla feels less confused now. She sees that her parents have backed off somewhat in their unrelenting emphasis on academic excellence. Yet, unresolved problems with authority figures still remain; she sometimes feels her parents act only in a bullying way and she still feels bridled by all the center's rules. She seems hopeful, however, about being able to endure the confinement of day care till reentry status.

Case No. 2: Gregory O'Higgins

Graduation from MCDC is a very special occasion, usually taking place twice a year with anywhere from one to four people graduating together. It is held during the evening in the church's gymnasium. Staff and parents organize the event; parents provide a buffet dinner that precedes the ceremony. Former program graduates and their parents are always invited. All current patients and their parents are required to attend. Some 200 to 250 people fill the hall to hear speeches given by staff, parents, siblings of the patient, and the patients themselves. Such occasions are seen as the culmination of treatment, accompanied by much applause and with many tears shed. Patients' families and staff commonly embrace each other, expressing complex feelings of loss, gratitude, and relief at the conclusion of therapy.

When Gregory was graduated it was a particularly emotion-filled experience. Gregory had been in the program for over three years, much longer than most graduating patients. Practically everyone at the ceremony knew him and his family owing to their long stay in the program. Gregory also had an older sister who had graduated from MCDC. Several counselors spoke of the tremendous metamorphosis that had taken place within him since Gregory first came to the center.

Upon entering the program at age fourteen Greg had been a very heavy drinker; he sometimes mixed alcohol with barbiturates. He was very depressed then, and had made several suicide gestures prior to intake. His counselors noted that during his first few months in the program he always kept his head down, never looked directly at anyone, and always spoke in a whisper.

Gregory came from a wealthy family; his father was the head of a very successful insurance agency, a family-run business, that had originally been established by Greg's grandfather. The O'Higgins family had a long history of prior mental health treatments. Mary O'Higgins, Greg's mother, had struggled with a long course of therapy and relapse for alcoholism. Greg's father, too, had received psychotherapy for many years.

When Greg first entered therapy at Manhasset it was apparent that he felt guilty about being a disappointment to his family. He had extremely low self-confidence and self-esteem. He ran away from the center on several occasions and had to spend much time out sitting on the prospect chair. In his sessions it became apparent that Greg fluctuated between feelings of anger toward his mother and her alcoholism for depriving him of a normal childhood and feelings of guilt for the trouble he himself caused. He sometimes even speculated that he alone had driven his mother to her initial bouts of heavy drinking and pill-taking. About two years after beginning therapy Greg had a big setback: he made a suicide attempt and had to be placed in a twenty-four hour care facility at a local psychiatric hospital. Shortly before his suicide attempt Greg's mother had undergone gall bladder surgery. Treatment records suggested a possible connection between his mother's surgery and Greg's sense of guilt that prompted the suicide attempt.

A month later Greg was released from the psychiatric facility and wanted to return to day treatment. Several staff members had reservations about his return, fearing a recurring suicide attempt, and questioning whether his current treatment regimen of antidepressant medication now made him inappropriate for the drug-free day center program. Given such reservations, he was nearly terminated from treatment. However, when the treatment staff fully reviewed the case, his abstinence from recreational drug use and his family's deep commitment to treatment led to his eventual reinstatement.

Greg's treatment dragged on beyond the normal two to two and a half year period to over three and a half years. He was kept in the reentry phase of treatment longer than most because he was younger and still required the support of the program. Two months prior to his graduation, the success of Greg's treatment was confirmed when his mother relapsed into alcoholism once again. The old Greg would have been inclined to act out his feelings of guilt and/or anger. This time, however, Greg was able to separate himself emotionally from his mother's relapse and was able to offer support to his family at this critical time. Greg also succeeded in becoming a good student at the local community college; he was accepted at a quality college which he planned to attend the next year. He also succeeded at work, and held a part-time job as night manager of a fast food restaurant.

At his graduation he spoke with poise and self-assurance; he was a greatly changed person from the former sheepish soul who stood in the corner and criticized himself.

Case No. 3: Frank Trivino

At age fifteen, when Frank was referred by his school to MCDC, he had established a reputation as a troublemaker. When Frank was caught selling pot to another student on school grounds, school officials threatened to report him to the police unless the Trivino family agreed to voluntarily withdraw Frank from school. The family agreed and entered Frank in drug rehabilitation treatment. In his first two years of high school Frank had been suspended on several occasions for his frequent fights with other students, high absenteeism, and failing grades. Frank also had a juvenile court record of several burglary and auto theft offenses. His drug consumption consisted chiefly of marijuana, cocaine, and alcohol several times weekly, although he would use any drug that was available.

Frank's early childhood was uneventful until the fifth grade when his mother divorced his father in order to live with another woman. Frank's father, a plumbing and heating contractor, struggled for six years to raise Frank and his older brother. During this period Frank's contact with his mother was sporadic. At the time of intake Frank's mother was living in a distant city and his father had remarried. The Trivino household then consisted of Mr. Trivino, his new wife, Frank, and his stepsister, Janine, an eight month old. Frank's eighteen year old brother had recently left home for college. Questions arose during the intake interviews regarding Frank's father and stepmother's ability to devote the time and attention necessary to participate in the program, as they were busily involved in caring for their young child. They insisted, however, that Frank's welfare was a top priority, and they vowed to do whatever necessary to assist in Frank's recovery.

Early sessions with Frank revealed that he felt a lot of hostility towards his father, mother, and stepmother. He remembered, as a small child, being unfavorably compared to his older brother who was always considered a model son—a good student and an industrious worker, who worked part-time in his father's business to save for college. By contrast, Frank was considered 'a bad seed,' always getting into trouble and doing the wrong things as a small child.

While Frank claimed that he liked his little stepsister, he had few positive things to say about his stepmother. Although she asserted her interest in Frank, he felt that she was impatient with him.

Frank's stay in the program was not very long, not quite six months. Although he had a positive relationship with his counselor and used his individual sessions constructively, Frank often flouted program rules and displayed antagonistic attitudes toward several staff members and patients almost regularly. Confrontation, by staff and his peers, did not produce much of a behavioral improvement. Frank ran away from the treatment center on several occasions. During treatment he continued to smoke marijuana. On many evenings his former friends left marijuana cigarettes outside his window, keeping him regularly supplied. When his parents were brought up to the center for his two separate suspensions, it became evident that they had neither the will nor the resources to closely watch over Frank so that he would comply with therapeutic expectations. After his second suspension Frank was terminated from treatment and referred to a residential facility.

When I interviewed Frank, nearly six years later, he was on the verge of being released from Phoenix House, a residential facility located in Northern Westchester County, about thirty miles north of New York City. He had been through several other programs since he left Manhasset. He remembered that the Manhasset program had been a great mistake for him at the time. He recalled that he was running wild during those days and felt the need to get away from his father and stepmother. He had the impression that they did not want him around; and they were unable to control him. He indicated that at that time he caused pain for everyone, including himself.

At twenty-one Frank had settled down and learned a trade, carpentry. In fact, he was the carpenter for Phoenix House, and did many of their carpentry jobs, not only at his own treatment facility, but at other Phoenix House Centers. He was looking forward to his imminent release from treatment, but he was somewhat apprehensive, too. He was concerned about how well he would do in aftercare, with only two group sessions a month. He had gotten used to talking about his feelings almost immediately, which was the way it was at Phoenix. Freedom from confinement was not an issue for Frank any longer; in reentry he was free to come and go as he pleased. He recognized that he had changed a great deal; he was not the same angry person he once was; now, instead, he accepted his parents and stepmother as they were. He said, "I don't have to prove anything to anyone else now, just myself."

These case studies make it clear that day treatment is not necessarily the most appropriate form of care for all types of problems of youth drug abuse. In the chapters that follow an attempt will be made to clarify which types of patients are the most and least appropriate for the day care modality, as well as to explore how effective this mode of care is in combating youth substance abuse problems. These, and other related issues, form the body of the ensuing analysis.

Note

1. Available information about Nassau County suggests that the treatment population is generally similar to the county population at large. Few blacks and Hispanics live in Nassau. According to information collected in U.S. Census in 1980 the black and Hispanic populations consisted of 6% and 3% respectively (Long Island Regional Planning Board, 1982).

Nassau is a wealthy county with a mean family income in 1979 of $37,744, making it number one nationally in effective buying income, according to Sales and Marketing Management's 1984 Survey of Buying Power. Half the county's families had incomes over $28,000 and only 5% had incomes below the poverty line in 1980. It contains relatively high percentages of managerial and professional employees—30%—of the sixteen and over male work force (Nassau County Planning Commission, 1985).

According to information provided by the Federation of Jewish Philanthropies and the Diocese of Rockville Center, 16% of all households in Nassau are Jewish and 47% Roman Catholic (Dunlap, 1982; Diocese of Rockville Center, 1986). Thus, the sample contained somewhat but not a great deal more Jews, Catholics, and managerial fathers than was noted in the population at large.

2

Methodological Considerations

Gathering the Data for This Study

The data for this study came from four different sources: (a) clinic files of sampled patients and their families; (b) interviews with a carefully selected subsample of patients collected three to eight years after their release from treatment; (c) urinalyses of specimens collected from this latter sample when former patients were interviewed; and (d) driving offense records for each interviewed former patient (among those possessing drivers' licenses) obtained from state departments of motor vehicles.

Coding Clinic Files

A two-thirds random sample of all patients entering day care treatment between 1977 and 1984 was selected for study. The treatment records of these patients were carefully examined and coded. Agency files for a given patient contained a number of reports and records that were generated during the course of treatment. Records usually contained a psychosocial evaluation of the adolescent client and their parents done by an agency social worker. Such psychosocial interviews were collected prior to admission to the program. In addition, a consulting psychiatrist usually did a psychiatric evaluation of the patient. CODAP drug use and agency application forms were also filled out by agency personnel when families were interviewed prior to admission. (CODAP stands for Client Oriented Data Acquisition Process. It is a federal government sponsored reporting system similar to Uniform Crime Reporting which requests all federally subsidized drug treatment programs to collect demographic and other data on all patients entering and terminating care.) Patient files also included copies of probation or court orders, school performance and aptitude test data, and copies of other relevant medical and psychiatric reports generated on clients before and during treatment.

During treatment, weekly and monthly reports were filed, recording each patient's attendance and participation in different treatment center activities.

Periodically, narrative reports and summaries were written by clinicians assessing the quality of a patient's participation and progress achieved in individual and group therapies. Similar reports were generated for parents and siblings involved in the treatment process. Clinic files also contained discharge information consisting of treatment summary statements, information on referrals made for patients, and CODAP drug use data at discharge.

After examining some dozen or more patient files a coding scheme was developed to enumerate the demographic and interactional elements of interest in this research. Then, files of sampled patients were examined and coded by the author. The coding scheme was revised on several occasions; as the list of codes were enlarged and modified, previously coded files were reexamined under revised coding categories. The finalized codebook is included in Appendix A. Coding extended from May, 1985 till October.

Selecting the Interview Sample

Among its many objectives, the basic experimental design of the follow-up research was to include a comparative analysis between those who remained in treatment at Manhasset for a year or more ("long-stay" patients) with those who withdrew after less than six months ("short-stay" patients). The specified subject population and time frame consisted of white male patients accepted for day care between 1977 and 1981.

My original intent was to obtain equal numbers of both long- and short-stay patients meeting those criteria that were included in the clinic file population. Yet it soon became apparent than many of Manhasset's short-stay patients had received an extensive variety of treatment experiences in many other drug programs and mental health facilities. It therefore became necessary to expand the sample of short-stay patients. Twice as many names of short-stay patients were ultimately selected to adjust for this attrition, thereby providing sufficient numbers of minimally treated individuals.

Owing to differences in refusal rates the size of the long-stay and short-stay subpopulations never quite matched up. This resulted in twenty long-stay patients, three-fourths of whom had completed the course of day care treatment. There were twenty-eight short-stay Manhasset patients; fourteen of whom had also obtained treatments elsewhere which did not extend beyond a total of six months; the remaining fourteen had spent extended time periods in treatment at a variety of different treatment facilities in addition to Manhasset day care. Such a sample seemed adequate for the research's exploratory purposes.

Interviewing Former Patients

Contacting and interviewing former patients proved to be the most laborious component of the data collection process. The accompanying interview schedule (Appendix B) was used in gathering the interview data. Questions spanned a range of behavioral and psychological issues pertaining both to the pretreatment conditions and social relationships of patients, their therapeutic experiences—both within and apart from the treatment facility under study, and post-treatment outcomes. The schedule was devised expressly for the present study. Many of the questions were adapted from interview instruments used in earlier follow-up studies of former drug patients, such as the Addiction Severity Index (McLellan, Luborsky, Woody and O'Brien, 1980), and other research instruments (Nehemkis, Macari, and Lettieri, 1976). Efforts were made to maximize overlap with existent instruments which would facilitate study comparisons.

Evaluating the effectiveness of day care treatment was a primary objective of the research. To do so it seemed most appropriate to compare those who spent a fairly substantial period of time in treatment with those who withdrew. Therefore, those who spent more than a year in day care treatment were contrasted to those who dropped out within the first six months.

Considering the research objectives it seemed advisable to limit attention to the white male population. White males predominated in the treatment population as a whole (68%), and the numbers of nonwhite and female clients in this particular program were so small that statistical analyses of nonwhites and women would have proved inadequate in assessing their experiences and outcomes.

Given existing gaps in knowledge about the longer-term effects of drug treatment it also seemed advantageous to confine attention to the patient population treated between 1977 and 1981. While it would have been desirable to extend the study back to the days of the program's inception, it was not possible to go back before 1977, because large numbers of treatment records from that period were no longer available. Confining the study to this five-year time frame also created a partial control for changes in program administration that had taken place since its initial foundation. The interviews of patients, therefore, occurred between three and eight years after their termination from day care treatment. The mean time since leaving the program was 6.06 years. Details of the sampling procedures for the interview subjects are given in a subsequent section.

Protecting the Rights of Former Patients   In a research project such as this, which deals with human subjects and inquires into the potentially damaging areas of drug use and criminal conduct, it is especially important to safeguard the rights of the population being studied. Before commencing the project, the Human Subjects Review Boards at Long Island Jewish Hospital and Nassau Community College examined and gave approval to a research proposal detailing the methods to be employed in gathering these data.

In addition, an application was made and obtained from the National Institute on Drug Abuse for a Confidentiality Certificate which afforded project research employees the privilege of protecting the privacy of their respondents

(Confidentiality Certificate No. DA-86-02). In the absence of such a certificate any research employee could be compelled to testify under penalty of court judgment if their information about a respondent was ever needed in a legal proceeding. This certificate protects respondents and research workers alike by providing immunity from prosecution against all subpoenas of research records. (Section 408 of Public Law 92-55 protects drug clients records and drug research against disclosure. Further protection is afforded under Section 872(c) of Title 21 of the United States Code, which vests authority in the Attorney General to give a grant of confidentiality to any drug research project. Section 0.100 of Title 28 of the code of Federal Regulations, as amended July 10, 1973 under 38 F. R. 18380-82, delegates this authority to the Administrator of the Drug Enforcement Administration of the Department of Justice.) Before any interview data was collected this waiver of immunity had been obtained.

Another potentially troublesome ethical issue surrounded contacting former patients years after they were in treatment. Embarrassment and condemnation could befall subjects if it were revealed that they had been former drug abuse patients. Any number of respondents might have married—or established other new or important relationships with others who did not know about their earlier problems of drug abuse—in the eight-year interval between their initial admission to treatment and this follow-up.

To avoid any possible embarrassment to subjects the following method was employed. Before conducting follow-up interviews a letter was sent to all sampled respondents at their last known address indicating that the hospital where they received treatment was making a study of some of its programs. The letters and envelopes from the hospital did not make reference to any specific programs or treatments that patients received. Nothing was included in the correspondence that could suggest that patients received drug abuse treatment. This was intended to spare subjects any difficulties, in the event the letter was opened by someone else. The letter asked for patients' cooperation in an evaluation of the hospital's programs being jointly made by the hospital and the author.

In the letters respondents were given assurances that all information they offered would be kept in strictest confidence. Any discussion of their behavior in all written reports would be presented only in statistical form. In addition, respondents were told that their cooperation was most important and potentially useful for improving the programs and services offered by the treatment facility. They were also told they would be contacted again in the near future. They were advised that the research was in compliance with federal informed consent regulations and that cooperation was entirely voluntary; they were free to refuse to cooperate with all or any part of the interview. (A copy of the letter is included in Appendix C.)

Shortly thereafter, interviewers called respondents at their last known telephone number to schedule appointments for future interviews at the respondent's home. All interviewers carefully heeded the explicit instruction given to avoid any reference that patients were former recipients of drug treatment. Only when interviewers spoke directly to former patients or their parents was it permissible to mention drug treatment.

Before beginning to collect the data, interviewers asked respondents to sign informed consent statements consisting of the following points: their cooperation with the research was entirely voluntary; they were free to answer as many or as few of the questions as they wanted; they were free to refuse the interview altogether; whether they cooperated or not with the study would in no way effect the likelihood of their receiving any future services from the treatment facility.

Interviewing Our Respondents

The interviews were conducted by a total of seven persons. In addition to the author, six other persons at different stages of professional accomplishment in the social service field also participated in this phase of the work. They included two administrative heads of social service programs, two graduate social work students completing Masters' degrees, and two mature adult students who were in the later stages of finishing undergraduate programs in social work. All these personnel were carefully trained in procedures for making respondent contacts and in administering the interview schedule.

Most of the interviews were conducted in respondents' (or parental) homes. Several were completed at the site of the treatment facility, a few others were conducted in restaurants or in the interviewer's automobile when opportunities for privacy were not available at a respondent's home. Nine of the forty-eight interviews (19%) were conducted over the telephone. Telephone interviews were administered when respondents lived more than seventy-five miles from Nassau County, or when respondents expressed reluctance to participate in a face-to-face interview, but were otherwise willing to cooperate.

Codebooks were created for coding the interview, urinalysis, and driver record data received for each respondent. The author coded all the interview and other data—transforming responses into numerical form—and logged them onto data files that could be read by SPSS on the Nassau Community College mainframe computer. Thereafter, the data was readily accessible to statistical analysis with SPSS.

Studying Drug Abuse: Special Problems

In research dealing with deviant behavior and with self-report information as the data base, questions can often be raised about validity and reliability. This concern becomes particularly important in research on substance abuse, where psychological denial of drug use as well as deliberate falsification could occur. Questions about the quality of the data might be raised at two points in the present study: pre-intake drug use and drug use at follow-up reported by former patients.

All pre-intake drug use information was collected by agency staff at the time of entry into Manhasset. One might wonder how much confidence can be placed in the reports given to agency personnel. Would it not have been better to have had trained interviewers—with specialized instruction in eliciting this sensitive information—to collect this data? One recent study suggests otherwise, indicating a close correspondence between the drug use information given to agency personnel as patients enter treatment and that given to trained interviewers (Kleinman, Wish, Deren, and Rainone, 1985). Thus, the study suggests that data gathered by agency personnel yields no less reliable and valid data than that obtained by employing trained interviewers throughout.

The second concern pertains to the self-report data furnished by respondents both at the time of intake and at follow-up—how reliable and valid is self-report data? Almost all past drug research has relied heavily upon such self-reported information. The present study is not unique in this respect; and whatever liabilities that may be inherent in dealing with such data must be acknowledged. However, the present study also included urinalysis, which provides an independent data source on recent drug use. While urine analysis adds additional depth to an understanding of drug use, it is no methodological panacea. More will be said shortly about the drug-use data obtained by self-reports and from urine analysis.

Problems Associated with Nonresponse

One of the most serious problems encountered in long-term follow-up studies is the possibility of bias due to high rates of nonresponse. Former patients who can be located with relative ease may be very different from those who are difficult to find. Such differences could be especially critical in studies like the present one, where deviant behavior and the failure to locate former clients could be closely intertwined. A high nonresponse rate could, indeed, call into question the representativeness of a drug abuse study's findings.

Earlier drug abuse follow-up studies have had greatly varying success in finding former patients years later at follow-up. Success rates range anywhere from 45% up to about 90%. Many factors seem to account for the variations in follow-up rates: the age and sex of former patients, the length of time since treatment, duration of treatment, type of drugs abused, and the kind of treatment given, among other factors. At the low end of the spectrum, Russe, McBride, McCoy, and Inciardi (1977) reported a 45% rate of participation among a sample of mostly younger patients who were originally treated for drug reactions in a metropolitan hospital emergency room in Miami, Florida. At the other end, Merton Hyman (1976) obtained much higher rates of cooperation, with 87% participation. Hyman's research involved interviewing a group of adult former alcoholics who were treated over a long duration, and followed up fifteen years later, in late middle and old age in suburban New Jersey (Hyman, 1976).

Given the similarities between our study population and those of the Russe group we anticipated some difficulty in tracking down former patients. In an effort to minimize the rate of nonresponse we applied the methods suggested by Goldstein et al. (1977) of relying upon formal and informal networks to help track down respondents. In most instances, besides home addresses and telephone numbers, clinic files included additional telephone numbers of parents at their places of employment and those of close relatives. Recent telephone directories (and those of adjacent counties) were also employed, which often proved helpful in locating respondents and their families who had moved. Additional address information was obtained from state departments of motor vehicles. (Most states will provide current license holder address data for a nomimal fee to those who furnish name and birth date information.) Each piece of information provided an additional opportunity to help locate respondents who could not be found at their previous addresses.

Exhaustive detective work often proved very helpful in making contact with those respondents that moved. In several cases a site visit to the former domicile of a respondent yielded valuable information from former neighbors. Two respondents were found when former neighbors gave interviewers information about a respondent's (or family member's) present residence.

Out of a total pool of seventy-three potential respondents, only nine (or 12%) ultimately proved to be unlocatable. An additional respondent had died during the interval between intake and follow-up; another respondent was under heavy antipsychotic medication in a psychiatric hospital and hence unable to participate. Of the remaining sixty-two potential respondents, forty-eight agreed to be interviewed, yielding an overall response rate of 77%. When one considers that most day care patients entered the Manhasset program involuntarily, this represents a rather high rate of cooperation. Table 2-1 lists all the most salient facts about the characteristics of the sample and the response rate.

Substantial differences in response-rate were noted between those patients who spent longer than a year in treatment at Manhasset and those who spent less than six months. The rate of cooperation among long-term Manhasset patients was 87%; for short-term patients the comparable figure was 72%. Evidently, the longer one's association with the program, the greater one's willingness to cooperate with the research.

In the present study parents were critical resources in gaining access to their adult or almost adult children. This was a double-edged sword. On the one hand, many respondents would not have been interviewed were it not for the fact that their parents provided us with current address information for their children who lived elsewhere. Some parents also were very influential in coaxing their child to participate. In several cases parental encouragement and insistence gained a respondents' participation that would not have been obtained otherwise.

Table 2-1.
Sample Characteristics

	Short-term patients	Long-term patients	Totals
Total potential respondents	48	25	73
Unlocatables	8	1	9
Hospitalized	0	1	1
Deceased	1	0	1
Refusals	11	3	14
Interviewed	28	20	48
Rate of cooperation (in percent)	72	87	77

Yet, the refusal rate was also increased because of the two-step process usually involved in trying to establish contact with former patients. In some instances parents functioned as gatekeepers, preventing interviewers from obtaining any additional information on the present whereabouts of their child. Some parents took initiatives to have their child not participate in the research; several parents spirited interviewers away rather abruptly, making it clear by their actions that they had not consulted with their child when they discouraged interviewers from making inquiries. There was at least one case where a parent's opposition to the research was instrumental in his son's refusal to be interviewed. In this case the father, an attorney, objected to the study as a matter of principle, indicating that it violated his rights to privacy. While his son showed some interest in participation, it was evident that as a member of his father's household, he was not inclined to go against his father's wishes.

Considering the refusal population the question arises whether former patient dysfunctionality is being minimized in this inquiry. Perhaps only those former patients who were functioning more effectively in society—whose drug abuse was less acute—were those who agreed to participate in the study. Of course, we have no way of knowing the full extent of dysfunctionality in the refusal population without current data on their responses. Yet, it would be a gross misunderstanding to assume that dysfunctionality was a primary component in a former patient's decision not to participate, since there is enough information on a sizable number of those who refused to be interviewed that indicates that many were functioning reasonably well. Their decisions not to be interviewed were in response to many factors; dysfunctionality probably played a minor part in their actions. Below are listed profiles of several respondents who refused to be interviewed. In each of the cases cited, and elsewhere throughout the text, significant personal details have been altered to assure respondents' (and nonrespondents') privacy.

Harvey Abrams (a pseudonym for the attorney's son mentioned above), for example, appeared to be functioning well at the time of follow-up. He had finished a four-year college degree in the years since completing the drug treatment program. With a partner he now runs a home improvements/carpentry business. He claimed to be uninvolved with drugs. His occasional social visits to the treatment facility to see former counselors and therapists provided credibility to his drug abstinence claims.

Barry Bornstein also refused to be interviewed, although he was extremely apologetic about his refusal. However, he said, very earnestly, that his short stay in the program was one of the worst moments in his life. He meant that his embarrassment and humiliation in being publicly recognized as a problem adolescent deeply disturbed him. He preferred not to talk about those times and wanted to distance himself as much as possible from that low point in his life. Barry still lives with his parents, in an affluent suburban community in northern New Jersey. He completed college and is now pursuing a graduate degree in accountancy.

Anthony Toscano also refused to be interviewed. He felt that his short stay in the program would make him a very uninteresting subject. He was particularly concerned about his file at the treatment center and whether it could possibly damage his present career choice of becoming an attorney. He is now a part-time law student at a metropolitan university and also works full-time at a clerical position in the legal field. He lives with his girlfriend in an inner city apartment, and claims to be free of drugs at the present time.

Frank Mahoney's mother said that it had been a gross error that her son was placed in the program at Manhasset. She, her husband, and Frank all deeply resented that Frank had had to go there, but he had been placed there at the insistence of the school guidance counselor and psychologist. According to Mrs. Mahoney the professionals could not understand that their son simply had a deep aversion to going to school. She acknowledged that Frank occasionally smoked marijuana, stating, however, that his use was never heavy, and that he never took any other drugs. His main problem had been truancy. Since he left school and the program, his mother felt he has been doing especially well. He still lived with his parents and has been working steadily for several years in an automobile repair shop as a mechanic. He rarely misses work; I was encouraged by his mother if I did not believe her, to speak to her son's employer for myself. However, given the family's resentment about the inappropriate placement of their son, his participation was extremely unlikely.

It became apparent after several broken appointments over a period of three months that David Gersten also refused to be interviewed. In the many discussions between himself and different interviewers, it was revealed that he runs and owns a very successful small business in installing automotive alarms; he also lived with a roommate. But little was learned about his current use of drugs. His main reason for not participating in the study was because of the anger he felt toward the program administration. After he had graduated from the program he was placed on "bad standing" because of his occasional marijuana use. (Bad standing is a status that program administration applies to some of its former patients. Persons so designated are considered to be harmful influences; current patients are prohibited from associating with those on bad standing; those so named are not permitted to visit the treatment facility or attend any of its social functions). He deeply resented this exclusionary treatment, thought it was very unfair, especially since in his estimation he was fully recovered.

Thus, from these few examples it is apparent that reasons varied greatly among those refusing to be interviewed. Dysfunctionality and drug abuse, obviously, were present in some of the cases, but it was not necessarily a predominating force. In most of the cases individuals were functioning very acceptably in society. At least four (out of fourteen) refusers indicated they had completed four-year college degrees during the post-treatment period, compared to two (out of a total of forty-eight) among all cooperating respondents. Although less was learned about their current drug use, heavy use patterns did not seem to be at all indicated by the information that was discerned from most nonrespondents. If there was any common element shared among many of those not participating it was resentment and anger toward the program and its administration, and to the compulsory forces dictating their participation in day care treatment. Nonrespondents also shared another common element, fear of jeopardizing the high status that some had attained since discharge.

These results are consistent with what has been found by other drug follow-up researchers. Merton Hyman, author of a fifteen-year follow-up study of a middle-aged and older former alcoholism treatment population in suburban New Jersey, found that his refusing subjects shared certain characteristics. He reported that:

On the whole refusers were better off than the others. All of them were either prosperous small businessmen or their wives were professional women. It seemed like high economic status made them skittish about being interviewed, not continuing drinking problems.[1]

Another follow-up research study, taken from a sample of former heroin users, found those refusing reinterview often included lower proportions of persons showing evidence of antisocial behavior (Kosten, Rounsaville, and Kleber, 1986).

Collecting the Urinalysis Data

After the interview was completed respondents were asked to provide a urine specimen. Shortly thereafter, the urine samples were given for laboratory analysis. Thin layer chromatography (TLC) effectively screens for about twenty substances in human urine; with even greater precision, enzyme immunoassay (EMIT) can detect the presence of opiates, PCP, cocaine, methadone, barbiturates, amphetamines, and marijuana. Gas chromatography is also used to confirm alcohol abuse. Of course, these tests vary in their effectiveness in confirming drug residues depending upon the type of drug consumed, its concentration at intake, and the time interval since ingestion. However, for most commonly abused drugs the tests provide validation of drug consumption for the previous twenty-four to thirty-six hours with anywhere from 80% to 95% accuracy (Wish et al., 1983; Chedekel and Patel, 1980).

Of the two commonly used drug screening tests, TLC and EMIT, each has its associated benefits and liabilities. The TLC can be administered fairly inexpensively, at less than five dollars per test. It also provides a very sensitive measure of hallucinogen and/or marijuana use. It has been shown to detect the presence of hallucinogens as long as a week after initial ingestion. Yet, its ability to detect the presence of cocaine and heroin is less reliable. One study showed it to yield much less accurate detection of opiates and cocaine than the more sensitive EMIT tests (Wish, Johnson, Strug, Chedekel, and Lipton, 1983). EMIT testing, however, is far more costly. Each particular drug must be tested for separately, and each test ranges from forty dollars per analysis. The tests are often used in conjunction with each other. First a TLC test is given; then, if positive results are shown, or if there is a supposition of a particular kind of abused drug, additional EMIT tests will be done.

Nevertheless, despite their proven utility the tests have been subject to criticism. False positive readings have been obtained among those who have been in marijuana smoke-filled environments, but who had not directly ingested the drug. False positive results have also been known to accompany recent consumption of commonly used substances such as quinine tonic soda, aspirin, and poppy seeds. Laboratory errors have also mistakenly attributed drug use to some individuals (Noble, 1986). Because of the body's rapid absorption of certain drugs, e.g. cocaine and alcohol, the tests are often unable to detect fairly recent consumption of these substances.

Given the limited funds available for the research and the particular interest in abuse of hallucinogenic drugs, we decided to rely exclusively on TLC testing, despite its attendant liabilities. After the interview was administered respondents were asked for a urine specimen.

The level of compliance in giving urine samples was mixed. Of the forty-eight respondents in the sample eleven could not comply because it was physically impossible to do so at the time of the interview; in these cases respondents were interviewed by telephone, or in the interviewer's automobile. In four other instances interviewers neglected to ask respondents for urine samples when conducting the interview. Thus, in a total of thirty-three interviews respondents were asked for a urine specimen. Overall compliance was less than satisfactory with only two-thirds (twenty-two respondents) cooperating. Apparently, after a usually long interview of between an hour and a half to two hours, and with no financial inducements, many respondents' willingness to offer further aid waned.

Yet, we found that program participation had a great deal to do with the willingness to give a urine sample. Striking differences in compliance were noted between long- and short-term Manhasset patients. All of the long-term Manhasset patients—whether they completed the course of treatment at Manhasset or not—furnished a urine specimen. This contrasted sharply with the 42% of short-stay respondents who complied with the same request. Evidently, long-term participation in a drug treatment program inspires a more readily accepting frame of mind to urine testing. About half of Manhasset's short-stay patients who were interviewed had also been treated in other drug and/or mental health programs. These respondents were more likely to provide urines than their untreated counterparts. Apparently, those who have had little exposure to the social worlds of drug treatment (and those who actively resisted them), showed little inclination to comply with any of their specific norms.

The results of the urine testing tended to confirm the self-report data. However, enough discrepancies existed between the different data sets to raise some serious questions about reliability. With only one exception, former patients claiming to be presently uninvolved with drugs were found to have negative TLC test results. In the one instance of a discrepancy, the subject, who admitted to only high alcohol use, tested positive on marijuana. This could indicate that he lied, or that the test gave a false positive report owing to any number of other causes.

Discrepancies were more frequently noted between those admitting to drug use whose TLC test results showed negative. Of the four whose test results showed positive, three admitted to using those drugs in the last two months. Yet, six additional respondents acknowledged use of marijuana and cocaine (the two most widely used illegal drugs among all respondents) where test results did not offer confirmation. In several of these cases the occasional use pattern of the respondent conforms to the range limits of TLC testing. In four cases respondents who reported frequent use patterns remained undetected by the tests. The acknowledged unreliability of the TLC test in identifying cocaine use can account for some of these instances where drug use was not disclosed by test results. Similarly, in four cases where respondents admitted to more than weekly use of marijuana, the test failed to identify their consumption.

Of course, one should be cautious in generalizing about urine testing from such a small sample. Nevertheless, if these findings suggest anything at all they suggest that TLC urine test results may tend to underreport drug use among former drug patient populations. The test is more likely to err on the conservative side in not detecting all admitted drug use. And owing to the possibility of false positive reports, great caution must be applied before using this test as a diagnostic and/or research instrument. Other recent evidence suggests that drug-testing laboratories may be reluctant to make assertions of drug consumption unless high levels of residues are noted. Otherwise, they may find themselves subjected to lawsuits (Altman, 1986).

At present, the limitations of the available drug tests are not well known among the public-at-large. The application of the tests may have a ring of scientific infallibility to many. Initially, their usage could inspire people to provide more truthful self-report information. Their administration—however it may infringe upon the civil liberties of citizens—may even influence people to reduce drug consumption. The recent application of drug testing to the American military has helped bring about marked reductions in marijuana use among military personnel (Halloran, 1986). Yet, in an environment where the tests are commonly applied, their acknowledged deficiencies will soon be realized, ultimately reducing any benefits that might come from them. Thus, such improvements in drug use knowledge are likely to be short-lived.

Today, increasing interest in employing drug testing can be found throughout all phases of government employment—in the military, for many groups of federal, state, and local government workers, for the police, fire fighters, and teachers. Some of the largest corporations are now insisting on drug testing of all new employees. Such companies include American Telephone and Telegraph, International Business Machines, Exxon, Lockheed Aircraft, Sherson Lehman Brothers, Federal Express, United Airlines, Hoffmann-La Roche, and Du Pont, among others (Kaufman, 1986). Professional and collegiate sports is another area where drug testing has now become well established. Yet, unless drug testing advocates are ready to bear the considerable expense for the most effective drug tests (such as careful EMIT screening and retesting)—under optimal laboratory conditions—they run the risk of creating a Kafkaesque nightmare for all workers. Given the current state of the art of drug testing, any mass testing scheme, with its attendant economizing measures, will be likely to result in drastically increased test errors.

The propriety of urine testing is a hotly debated subject today. The controversy is one that demands our most considered attention. If evidence continues to mount against the tests, showing their unreliable and/or invalid results, then this should be a strong point against any widening application of such testing.

Collecting Driver License Data on the Respondents

Most states for a nominal fee (usually $2.00) provide copies of the abstract of any driver who is licensed to drive in that state. Abstracts contain the address, birth date, driving restrictions, license expiration information and lists motor vehicle offenses of license holders, reported accidents and injuries, license suspensions, and drug-related driving charges.

Copies of these records were requested for each of the forty-eight respondents in the follow-up study. Thirty-six of our forty-eight respondents (75%)

had drivers licenses in New York, Florida, and Pennsylvania. These data were coded and analyzed, forming another part of this research.

Note

1. Merton Hyman, personal communication, October, 1986.

3

Analysis of Program Records: Social Factors Affecting the Completion of Day Care Treatment

One of the more important goals of the research was to identify the social characteristics associated with completing day care treatment. This information has multifold practical applications to drug abuse treatment administrators for better understanding which populations will be inclined to seek and complete their programs, as well as those likely to avert and withdraw from treatment. Such knowledge can be useful for better identifying which groups and individuals will require special outreach efforts and "fine tuning" of program requirements, to promote a fuller utilization of treatment resources.

In the absence of any available statistics summarizing the social characteristics of those admitted to adolescent day treatment programs nationally, we had no way of gauging whether the Manhasset population typified most of such programs. Certainly the high numbers of Jewish, Italian, and affluent members found in Nassau County made it somewhat unique in at least these aspects. Yet, Manhasset's population represented a good beginning point for establishing baseline data on those persons and families who are best able to use the day care treatment modality.

The course of treatment was intended to last for an approximately two-year period at this day care program. In the two-thirds random sample of all those admitted for treatment between 1977 and 1984 those who completed the program spent from a minimum duration of nineteen months to a maximum of thirty-nine months in treatment.

But only 14% of those admitted to the program completed the course of day care treatment. Hence it was important to discover what factors distinguished those who completed treatment from those who left prematurely.[1]

Age as a Factor Influencing Treatment Success

Most of the incoming patient population were concentrated in the fourteen to sixteen year age group (77%), with the remainder thirteen years old or

Table 3-1.
Completion of Treatment by Age (frequencies in parentheses)

	AGE 14 and younger	15	16 and Older
COMPLETED TREATMENT			
Completed	4% (2)	12% (6)	20% (16)
Withdrew	96% (42)	88% (44)	80% (65)
Column totals	(44)	(50)	(81)

younger (6%) or seventeen and older (17%). The youngest admitted patient was twelve years old and the oldest was 20. Those who were disparate in age from the majority of the treatment population tended to be among those more likely to withdraw. Since the program heavily relied on peer pressure to achieve its objectives, those who were extremely different in age from the rest were more likely to feel anomalous from other members of their treatment groups. Their outsider status probably added to any adjustment difficulties they may have encountered in getting treatment.

A very clear pattern was also noted between younger and older patients in completing treatment. Older patients were significantly more likely to finish treatment. Among those aged fourteen and younger only 4% completed treatment, compared with 20% among the sixteen and over population. This difference was statistically significant at the .05 level using the Chi Square test.

A related pattern was found in the educational attainments of the sample. Among those who had completed the eighth grade or less only 9% had completed the program, in comparison with 19% among those finishing tenth grade or higher education.

These age trends are somewhat at odds with the findings obtained in the DARP follow-up study (Sells and Simpson, 1979). In that comprehensive study of all major treatment modalities, Sells and Simpson found somewhat more favorable treatment outcomes among the younger patients. Yet, in that study the age ranks were grouped much differently than at present; the eighteen-year-old and younger population were compared with those first entering treatments during adulthood.

These results are consistent with the view that as these youngsters move into later adolescence they attain higher levels of emotional maturity which help them to meet the challenges of program expectations. However, it was not completely clear whether age itself was linked with treatment completion, or whether older patients—who already had treatment prior to entering Manhasset—were more likely to complete because of this experience, rather than age.

We cross-tabulated whether one had any prior mental health or drug care elsewhere (before enrolling for care at MCDC) with program completion at Manhasset. The analysis showed little differences in completion rates among the two populations: 13% among those with previous treatment experience compared with 17% whose participation at Manhasset was their first therapeutic experience. Those who had been in residential drug treatment programs before entering Manhasset were no more likely to complete the day care program than those who had not: 18% as compared to 14%.

The importance of age in completing treatment was manifested in still another way. Those who began using drugs at earlier ages were less likely to finish treatment, as compared to those starting drug use later in life. For those trying drugs before age thirteen, only 11% completed the program. This compared with 33% among those fifteen or older. This was significant at the .05 level with Chi Square. This is corroborated by Maddux and Desmond's (1981) evidence in their follow-up study of opioid abusers in Texas.

Thus, when patients enter treatment as older teenagers and when they start abusing drugs at later ages, appear to be linked with their success in getting day care treatment.

Ethno-religious Identification as a Predictor of Treatment Outcome

Another meaningful correlate of treatment completion was ethnoreligious identification. The completion rate for Jews was much higher than for any of the other groups; 28% of the Jewish patients completed the program as compared with 17% of Protestant patients and only 6% of the Catholics. This difference was significant at the .001 level with Chi Square.

In an attempt to further differentiate the largest religious subgroup of Catholics, they were further subdivided into four subgroups: Irish, Italians, Hispanic, and others. These designations were assigned on the basis of the ethnic origins information included in the files. It was also assigned by a coding of surnames. Names like 'Gonzalez' were assigned to the Hispanic designation, 'O'Malley' to the Irish, 'Toscano' to the Italian, etc. Any ambiguous names were assigned to the residual category of Other Catholics. Since of all ninety-eight Catholics in the sample only six had completed the program, completion could not be used as a criterion for looking at differences among Catholics. Instead, we looked at the number of months each ethnic group of Catholics remained in treatment. A very interesting pattern emerged. Italian patients tended to drop out from treatment the earliest, while Irish patients were inclined to withdraw last. Table 3-2 shows the pattern for each of the four subgroups.

One may speculate that Italian families are inclined to experience conflict with the treatment center soon after initiating treatment, often causing these

Table 3-2.
Time in Treatment by Ethnic Affiliation among Catholics
(frequencies in parentheses)

| | ETHNIC AFFILIATION | | | |
	Italian	Irish	Hispanic	Other
MONTHS IN TREATMENT				
6 months or less	65% (15)	40% (10)	50% (4)	41% (20)
7 to 12 months	17% (4)	16% (4)	38% (3)	29% (14)
Over a year	17% (4)	44% (11)	13% (1)	31% (15)
Column totals	(23)	(25)	(8)	(49)

families to terminate their contact with the center. A potential source of conflict could arise as the treatment center challenges the pattern of reliance upon familial authority for resolving personal problems shared by many Italian-Americans. Contrastingly, in the Irish-American home, efforts are made to abide by treatment rules and regulations, although, as the course of treatment proceeds, differences between the family and the treatment center become more apparent, causing families to withdraw and leading professional staff to recognize that little progress was actually occurring.

These results should not be entirely surprising. This interpretation of the data is consistent with evidence collected by other investigators in a variety of other kinds of treatment settings. The psychotherapeutic seeking inclinations of Jews—their inclinations both to seek and successfully utilize therapies—has been documented by several investigators (Srole et al., 1962; Hollingshead and Redlich, 1958). Other researchers have found Italians to be reluctant to utilize mental health facilities and other social support services and more inclined to rely on their families for aid (Rabkin and Struening, 1976). In his study of Italians in Greenwich Village, Tricarico (1984) noted that when adolescents were found to have substance abuse problems, those drawing upon resources outside the family turned to family physicians rather than local community substance abuse programs. Others studies suggest that if professional caretakers are to succeed in providing services to Italian families they will need to surmount the barriers that are often erected between these families and the outside world, (Zola, 1966; Zborowski, 1969).

According to Monica McGoldrick (1982), the Irish tend to be rebellious in family therapy, while at the same time they tend to be compliant in accepting authoritarian structures. Although disinclined to seek mental health therapies, they are overrepresented among psychiatric patients (Roberts and Myers, 1954; Rabkin and Struening, 1976; Murphy, 1975). Several other studies document the external compliance among Irish patients while receiving mental

Table 3-3.
Completion of Treatment by Father's Occupational Status
(frequencies in parentheses)

| | FATHER'S OCCUPATIONAL STATUS | | |
	Managerial/ Professional	Low White Collar	Blue Collar
COMPLETED TREATMENT			
Completed	22% (15)	9% (3)	5% (1)
Withdrew	78% (53)	91% (48)	95% (22)
Column totals	(68)	(73)	(23)

health treatments (Zborowski, 1969; Zola, 1966; Sanua, 1960). Yet, as treatment progresses conflicts often arise when compliance is not linked with emotional response and the motivation to change behavior (Zborowski, 1969; McGoldrick, 1982). These patterns are all consistent with our findings that Irish patients remained for relatively long periods in treatment, but eventually dropped out.

Parental Characteristics

Father's occupational status was another variable linked with completing treatment. Twenty-two percent of managerial/professional/proprietor fathers had children who were able to successfully use the program. This compared to 9% among lower level white-collar fathers and 5% among all fathers in blue collar occupations. This was significant at the .05 level of significance.

These findings should come as no surprise. Many studies have demonstrated the greater receptivity of higher status patients to completing mental health treatments. (Hollingshead and Redlich, 1958; Srole et al., 1962; Dohrenwend and Dohrenwend, 1969). The more ample resources of the higher classes, their greater self-confidence and facility in dealing with professional staff, their proclivity for inspiring acceptance and admiration among treatment personnel all serve to promote their child's successful movement through programs such as the Manhasset Community Day Center.

Parental drug abuse and prior experience of treatment seemed to be linked with the day care outcomes of their children. A trend was noted among the fathers with a history of substance abuse and their child's treatment completion status. Only 8% of fathers with a history of substance abuse had children who completed the course of treatment, while 17% of moderate drinking fathers' children completed care. This difference approached, but fell short of, statistical significance at the .05 level with Chi Square. No such similar pat-

Table 3-4.
Completion of Treatment by Parental Substance Abuse
(frequencies in parentheses)

	FATHER'S DRUG ABUSE		MOTHER'S DRUG ABUSE*	
	Abuse History	Moderate Drinker	Abuse History	Moderate Drinker
COMPLETED TREATMENT				
Completed	8% (4)	17% (11)	16% (4)	13% (10)
Withdrew	92% (47)	83% (53)	84% (21)	87% (67)
Column totals	(51)	(64)	(25)	(77)

*Psychosocial evaluations contained information on family histories of substance abuse. In this analysis parents with histories of alcohol and drug abuse were compared with others described as moderate drinkers.

tern seemed to prevail for the mothers. For mothers, the respective figures were as follows: 16% completion rate for those with substance-abusing mothers, compared with 13% among those whose mothers were only moderate drinkers. Table 3-4 displays the cross-tabulation results of parental substance abuse and program completion.

Does the fact that one's parents have sought treatment for themselves affect a child's likelihood of staying in treatment? The results suggested that when parents received mental health treatment for themselves there was a greater chance of their child's completion of day care. Parents receiving treatment were most likely to have a child complete treatment. Well and untreated parents formed an intermediate category. The group least likely to have a child finish day care consisted of parents who were described as having psychological problems of various sorts but who remained untreated. Here, mothers' experiences of receiving prior care seemed to be closely linked to their child's accepting care. Twenty-three percent of mothers with a history of mental health problems and treatment had children finishing day care. This contrasted to 10% among the mothers who were reportedly well and had not received any mental health treatment. None of the mothers who had problems and remained untreated had children finishing the program. These differences were significant with Chi Square at the .01 level. For fathers, the trend was similar and approached statistical significance, but the differences were less profound. The respective figures for fathers who had problems and got care was 20%; 14% among well fathers, and 4% among the untreated. Tables 3-5 and 3-6 display the trends linking program completion and parental experiences of mental health treatment.

Table 3-5.
Completion of Treatment by Mother's Mental Health Care
(frequencies in parentheses)

| | MOTHER'S MENTAL HEALTH PROBLEMS AND CARE | | |
	Had problems received care	Well untreated	Had problems, no care
COMPLETED TREATMENT			
Completed	24% (15)	10% (9)	0% (0)
Withdrew	76% (48)	90% (80)	100% (16)
Column totals	(63)	(89)	(16)

Patient Characteristics

Sex Differences

Although other researchers (DeLeon, 1984) have found females to be more likely to complete drug treatment programs, our clinic data showed no sex differences. Fourteen percent of males and 12% of females completed the course of treatment at Manhasset.

Prior Treatment Experiences

Many drug treatment specialists believe that, in order to effectively participate in treatment, a backlog of previous treatment experiences is helpful or even mandatory. However, our findings did not provide confirmation for this belief in the case of adolescent drug abusers. As mentioned above, the results

Table 3-6.
Completion of Treatment by Father's Mental Health Care
(frequencies in parentheses)

| | FATHER'S MENTAL HEALTH PROBLEMS AND CARE | | |
	Had problems received care	Well untreated	Had problems, no care
COMPLETED TREATMENT			
Completed	20% (8)	14% (13)	4% (1)
Withdrew	80% (32)	86% (80)	96% (23)
Column totals	(40)	(93)	(24)

showed little differences in the completion rates between those with previous treatment experiences and the uninitiated: 13% finished the program among those with previous mental health or drug treatment experiences compared to 17% among the novices. The data suggests that parental treatment experience is a far more potent force for predicting adolescents' treatment outcomes, especially that of the patient's mother.

Prior Criminality

Consistent with the findings of other researchers, we found a trend showing those entering treatment with more serious criminal records more likely to withdraw prematurely (Clayton, 1980; Jessor and Jessor, 1977). Only 12% of those committing prior serious crimes (e.g., burglary, auto theft, etc.) finished the program, compared with 25% of those with no past criminal activities. Those with only juvenile status offense records represented an intermediate group, with 15% of this subgroup completing the program. Although in the predicted direction, these differences fell somewhat short of statistical significance with Chi Square ($p = .15$).

Depression

Previous researchers have documented the role of depression in precipitating and sustaining teenage drug abuse (Parry et al., 1974; Paton et al., 1977). In the present investigation depression was found to be an important obstacle for receiving professional help. All adolescent patients were evaluated by a psychiatrist as part of the intake process. Those described as moderately or seriously depressed at intake were found to be much less likely to complete treatment. Only 6% of those described as depressed completed the program, as compared to 21% of those who were not regarded as having such difficulties. These differences were statistically significant at the .004 level with Chi Square. Table 3-7 shows the relationship between depression and program completion.

Self-Referral

Other studies have documented self-referral to be an important correlate of treatment outcome (Stimmel et al., 1978). Self-referred patients and families have been found to be more likely to succeed than those mandated to participate by the courts or other outside agencies. Our data showed a trend consistent with such findings. Twenty-six percent of self-referred patients completed treatment, as compared to 13% among those referred to the program by the courts and 11% among those referred by other social agencies. These differences approached, but fell short of, statistical significance at the .05 level ($p = .073$).

Table 3-7.
Completion of Treatment by Patient's Psychological State
(frequencies in parentheses)

| | PATIENT'S PSYCHOLOGICAL STATE AT INTAKE | |
	Depressed	Not Depressed
COMPLETED TREATMENT		
Completed	6% (5)	21% (19)
Withdrew	94% (76)	79% (70)
Column totals	(81)	(89)

Family Structure/Divorce

Other factors suspected of having linkages to treatment outcomes were also examined. Whether adolescents lived with both parents, or if they lived in an attenuated household (with one parent), or if they lived in a reconstituted family (with a parent and stepparent) seemed to be unrelated to treatment outcomes. Fifteen percent of those living with both parents completed treatment, compared to 13% in one parent households and 22% living with parent and stepparents.

Family Structure/Siblings

When the child was the only child living at home there was a greater likelihood of his/her remaining in treatment, compared with other children living in larger households. Of those children who were the only child living at home at the time of their initiation into treatment, 21% finished it, as compared to 12% who were members of larger families. Although a trend seemed apparent, the differences were not close to attaining statistical significance at the .05 level. However, when the data for only child living at home was cross-tabulated with the number of months they remained in treatment, a statistically significant relationship was noted ($p < .002$). It may well be that having only one child living at home at the time of participation might have made it somewhat easier for families to comply with program expectations.

Sibling order per se was apparently unrelated. Treatment completion rates were substantially alike among only, eldest, youngest, and middle children. However, those patients who had older brothers were less likely to finish treatment compared to all other types of sibling/age relationships. Seventeen percent of those without older brothers completed treatment as contrasted to 6% among those with older brothers; this was significant with Chi Square at the .05 level of significance. The impact of adoption on treatment outcome was

Table 3-8.
Completion of Treatment by Substance Abuse of Patient's Siblings
(frequencies in parentheses)

| | HAD SIBLINGS THAT ABUSED DRUGS | |
	With Sib Drug Abusers	Without Sib Abusers
COMPLETED TREATMENT		
Completed	17% (10)	13% (13)
Withdrew	83% (50)	87% (91)
Column totals	(60)	(104)

also explored, and we found adopted children to be no less or more likely to complete the program compared to those growing up with their natural parents.

If a patient had another sibling under care at the program, this was linked with success, although it was only marginally significant ($p = .15$). Twenty-four percent of those with other siblings in treatment at Manhasset completed the program, as compared with 12% among those without siblings in treatment. It was probably easier for families to accommodate treatment expectations with several of their children in the program at the same time. Familiarity with program requirements was likely to be greater with several children under care. Also, rule compliance difficulties arising from denying opportunities to the child in treatment that were available to other family members were lessened.

Other research has found that the drug-taking of siblings often prompts similar behavior for other children in a family (McCaul et al., 1982). On the basis of such evidence one might have anticipated that having a sibling with a history of drug abuse would have a negative effect on a child's treatment. However, the data did not show such a relationship, as demonstrated in Table 3-8. Seventeen percent of those having a sibling with a substance abuse history finished the program, as compared to 13% among those who were the only children in their families known to be drug involved.

Patterns of Prior Drug Abuse

We also examined for relationships between the patterns of drug abuse and treatment outcomes. Here, results showed few associations. Those whose drug abuse was confined to alcohol and/or marijuana use were no more or less likely to finish treatment than those using harder drugs. The number of abused drugs at intake was also unrelated to program completion. See Table 3-9

Table 3-9.
Completion of Treatment by Kind of Substance Abuse Problem
(frequencies in parentheses)

| | NO. OF DRUGS ABUSED | | | HARD DRUG ABUSE | |
	(1)	(2)	(3)	Hard	Soft only
COMPLETED TREATMENT					
Completed	11 (2)	11 (10)	19 (12)	15% (22)	8% (2)
Withdrew	89 (17)	89 (79)	81 (53)	85% (128)	92% (23)
Column totals	(19)	(89)	(65)	(150)	(45)

which shows the cross-tabulation between the abuse of hard drugs, the number of drugs abused, and completing day care treatment. None were statistically significant.

These findings seem to be at odds with previous research which has shown higher abuse patterns linked with withdrawals from treatment (Biase and Hijazi, 1977). Future research on day care will need to further explore the patterns of prior drug use and treatment completion.

In the treatment population drug abuse extended to include a wide variety of drugs, although several drugs were rarely abused by this treatment population: heroin and inhalants (only three respondents reported abusing heroin and inhalants); methadone and other opiates were reportedly not used by any of these patients. Alcohol, marijuana, cocaine, barbiturates, sedatives, and hallucinogens were most commonly consumed. None of these drug use patterns were linked to treatment outcomes except for barbiturate use. Barbiturate abusers were more likely to finish the program (25%) compared to those never abusing this drug (9%). What accounts for this particular pattern remains unclear.

Family Participation and Treatment Success:
A Circular Process

As indicated in the introductory chapter, patients' families were generally expected to play a pivotal role in the treatment process. Parents were expected to attend weekly therapy sessions at the treatment center; they were obliged to participate in carpooling and weekend chaperoning arrangements; in addition to a variety of other requirements, they were expected to abstain from drug use while their child was in treatment. Parents who were unwilling to comply with program expectations inevitably clashed with staff, usually resulting in the family's termination, unless parents indicated their resolve to comply with the center's therapeutic requirements.

Treatment records were established and maintained for each patient's parents. Periodic entries were made noting parental attendance, and behavior and attitudes shown to treatment staff. The attitudes and actions of parents inspired self-fulfilling prophesies among professional staff which affected treatment outcomes. When parents attended treatment sessions regularly and were supportive of the treatment regime, they were perceived by staff as contributing to treatment progress. And correlatively, when parents attended sessions sporadically and frequently violated treatment rules, they were viewed by staff as undermining their child's treatment at the center.

These staff beliefs were supported by the treatment reports data. There were no recorded cases of patients who completed treatment whose mother or father had attended fewer than forty-five treatment sessions. Contrastingly, among withdrawing patients no more than 15% of mothers and 10% of fathers had attended forty-five or more parent treatment sessions. Thus, parental participation was an indispensable requirement for program completion.

When children resided with both parents case records were coded in terms of whether both parents were equally involved in their child's treatment or whether one parent was more involved than the other, and if neither parent seemed concerned about the treatment. Mutual parental concern was clearly linked to treatment success. Thirty-three percent of equally involved parents had children finishing treatment, compared to 10% where only fathers were reportedly involved, and 5% among mother-involved families, and none of the neither-involved parents had children completing treatment. The differences were statistically significant with Chi Square at the .001 level. Table 3-10 displays the relationship between parental involvements and program completion. Apparently, when staff members found parental involvement to be nonexistent for both parents, and wrote it up in their official treatment progress reports, this was a prelude to program termination.

Interestingly, the trends demonstrating the importance of parental mutuality were also reflected in the family intake reports. In the ninety cases where these matters were discussed, it was noted that when parents were described as sharing equally in disciplining their child, half of these children completed treatment. This contrasted with 10% where mothers served as disciplinarians, and 16% where fathers functioned as primary disciplinary agents. This trend was statistically significant with Chi Square at the .002 level.

Parental cooperation was closely linked to treatment success. Thirty-one percent of the families where both parents were described as being cooperative during treatment had children who finished the program. This contrasted to none of the families completing treatment where only one parent cooperated and where neither cooperated, which also proved significant at the .001 level. Again, when clinicians recognized that parents were behaving uncooperatively it was only a matter of time before the adolescent patient and parents were terminated from this particular treatment program.

Treatment reports contained information about the psychological state of parents during treatment; reports mentioned some parents as being angry and

Table 3-10.
Completion of Treatment by Parental Mutual Involvement
(frequencies in parentheses)

| | PARENTAL MUTUAL INVOLVEMENT IN TREATMENT | | | |
	Mutual Involvement	Father more than mother	Mother more than father	Neither involved
COMPLETED TREATMENT				
Completed	33% (16)	10% (1)	5% (2)	0% (0)
Withdrew	67% (33)	90% (9)	95% (42)	100% (25)
Column totals	(49)	(10)	(44)	(25)

hostile, withdrawn, anxious, hysterical, guilt ridden, defensive, etc. Other reports described parental behavior as being devoid of psychopathological aspects. "Parent A showed insight into her feelings of loss and grief over the death of her father." When reports indicated psychopathology in parents fewer had children who successfully concluded treatment. Only 6% of mothers with psychological problems and 5% of like fathers had children completing care. This contrasted to 21% and 22% among symptom-free mothers and fathers whose children completed treatment. These differences were also significant at the .001 level with the Chi square statistic.

The program administration emphasized parental abstinence from drugs and alcohol while they had a child in treatment at the program. There were numerous incidents during the course of the program's history where a parent's continued drug use brought about the family's termination from the program. Yet, analysis of treatment records revealed that the rule of abstinence was not universally applied, and there were several exceptions where parental drug use did not result in automatic program termination. Usually these occasions occurred later during the course of treatment, when the adolescent patient had been making obvious progress in combatting his own problems of drug abuse.

In most instances of heavy parental drug abuse this would be recognized by other family members and would eventually become a treatment issue. With program completion as the dependent variable we cross-tabulated the cases where parental drug use arose as a issue during treatment and those cases where parents apparently refrained from drug-taking. The data showed no significant differences or trends between those drug abstinent and drug involved parents with 13% and 16% of both groups respectively completing treatment. On the basis of these findings it appears that program administration may have overemphasized the importance of parental abstinence for successfully completing treatment for teenage abuse.

Behavior during Treatment and Treatment Outcome

Family Conflict

Case records included much information about patients and their families behavior during treatment. Instances of family conflict occurred often enough in some families that staff members enumerated such actions in their periodic treatment commentaries. In half of the families where treatment notes never mentioned any family conflict children completed the course of treatment; this contrasted to only 9% completing care in conflict-resident households. This difference was significant at the .001 level. None of the families where physical conflict took place between family members had children completing treatment, as compared to 18% in physical conflict-absent homes. This difference was significant at the .02 level with the familiar Chi Square statistic.

Criminality and Mental Health

Criminality and mental health problems also were obstacles in the path to receiving drug abuse treatment. None of the patients engaging in any criminal activities during the course of their care completed treatment, and none of the those attempting suicide or showing other signs of serious depression were recognized as successfully completing care. This was contrasted to 18% completing in crime and depression-absent patients. Those completing the course of treatment had amassed treatment records indicating fewer drug abuse incidents, fewer acts of other rule-violating conduct, and more frequent reports acknowledging their cooperation. Thus, the conventional behavior and drug abstinent record that patients and their parents established at the center generated its own confirmation, with staff ultimately deeming a patient (and family) worthy of graduation and completion of treatment.

Summary and Conclusions

This research has attempted to enlarge the understanding of how day care rehabilitations are brought about by identifying some of the social correlates associated with the completion of treatment. To a large extent, in the program studied we noted that program completion signified the conferring of a reward for a history of compliant and drug-free behavior. Patients who were allowed to graduate from the program had long demonstrated their abstinence in periodic urine testing and in the many counseling and other encounters held with professional staff. They were acting conventionally in a variety of ways: job-holding and/or going to school, refraining from criminal activities, and establishing more harmonious relationships both with the outside world and with their families. Patients appeared to be functioning appropriately; they looked and acted "cured" to treatment personnel. Treatment completion was a status recognizing what had already become a well established social fact among members of the treatment community. Patients (and their families) were now perceived as "better" and no longer in need of the treatment facility's services.

As the research has demonstrated, getting to that point is a result of a complex array of causes and their interaction. The disposition of the entering patient—their determination and other strengths—had a great bearing on the treatment outcome. It was also a result of the patient's family, their motivations, resources, and perseverance in enduring a long course of demanding therapeutic interventions. In addition, it was also the product of meanings shared and transmitted between the patient's family and the treatment staff. Communication between these groups established a sense of worth about the therapeutic enterprise among patients and their families. At the same time it engendered a sense of propriety shared by treatment staff that patients had become ready for treatment completion or graduation.

This data established that older adolescent patients were more likely to complete the program than younger ones. Self-referred patients also tended to be more likely to meet the program demands than those referred by the courts and other outside social agencies; this trend approached but did not attain statistical significance at the .05 level. Program completers were less likely to be diagnosed as depressed at intake.

Parental characteristics and interaction constituted another array of factors which also impacted upon treatment outcomes. Parents of higher occupational rank, who had received mental health care for themselves, and of Jewish ethnicity appeared to possess useful strengths for meeting program challenges.

Parents of completing patients must inevitably attend many therapeutic sessions where they evince a pattern of regular attendance with cooperative inclinations. The pattern of spouse mutuality in dealing with their children's needs, as it existed preceding and during treatment, seemed to be another asset for successfully getting through this form of treatment. While parents with the above characteristics possessed resources that helped them to endure the rigors inherent in this form of care, these attributes also helped project positive images to professional staff about the family and patient's commitments to treatment. Parents that were unwilling and/or unable to show involvement in program endeavors, those behaving in a manner regarded by staff as uncooperative, inevitably withdrew from this form of care.

The results also demonstrated that certain family structural arrangements facilitated or impeded program completion. Three particular types of family structures were linked with remaining in treatment longer or finishing: (1) children who were the only children living at home in their families; (2) those having siblings that had been in treatment at the program, and (3) those without older brothers.

One might have expected parents of unbroken marriages to have an easier time at meeting treatment goals compared to the single parent or the parent in a reconstituted marriage. It seems plausible to anticipate that these parents might possess greater personal resources and commitments to the patient than the other groups of parents, but the results showed otherwise. Parents of intact marriages, single parents, and parents in reconstituted marriages all achieved substantially similar rates of day care completion.

It is important to recognize that although particular identifiable social characteristics were found to be associated with treatment completion, the relations were far from perfect. While patients of certain class and ethnic affiliations were more inclined to withdraw from treatment programs than others, there are many who would be able to utilize and benefit from treatment if given the appropriate kinds of inducements and incentives. It is incumbent upon program administrators to recognize that certain groups and individuals may require special additional kinds of care and cultivating efforts if they are to take advantage of available programs. Programs will have to be tailored to meet the diverse sets of needs, abilities, and handicaps that patients present when entering treatment. It represents a creative challenge to program administration of immense proportions to expand program utilization without diluting basic therapeutic principles.

As more is learned about the populations attracted and repelled by different treatment programs administrators will gain considerably. Such information will enhance successes in referring unworkable cases to alternative treatment approaches; it can also encourage a reevaluation and revision of therapeutic requirements maximizing the numbers of persons served.

This chapter has attempted to establish a beginning point toward better understanding how day care programs work at helping polydrug abusing adolescents and those inclined to use this treatment modality. More research will be needed to further delineate the social characteristics linked with differing adolescent outpatient drug abuse treatments.·

Note

1. In the analysis treatment completion served as the primary dependent variable. Time in treatment was also used as a secondary dependent variable. (Those spending a year or more under care were contrasted with the others who remained in treatment less than a year.) This conception seemed to make the most sense theoretically, since completing treatment represented a social recognition of a patient's improvement or cure, while time in treatment did not. Appendix D displays the Chi Square values and significance levels for each of the independent variables appearing in the analysis with the dependent variables. The soon to be discussed patterns of association were generally consistent with both of the dependent variables. As expected, treatment completion proved to be the most responsive dependent variable. There were also several instances where a relationship did not show up with treatment completion but did with time in treatment; most of these instances are mentioned in the text.

4

Post-treatment Adaptations: Comparisons between Short-term and Long-term Patients

During the many days I spent at the Manhasset drug treatment center examining patient files, I was often drawn into conversations about the research by a number of the counselors and social workers. They were deeply interested in the follow-up part of the study—and in knowing what had happened to many of their former patients since treatment. I was often advised by several long-time workers to make it a point to interview Harold Rosen (a pseudonym). Harold was respected by many staff as one of MCDC's success stories. He made frequent visits to the center to chat with his former counselors. When he came by he gave every indication of being free of drug problems and was reportedly well adjusted psychologically. He was said to be doing very well financially, happily married and now living in a luxurious home in the affluent suburban community of Great Neck. For these workers, Harold epitomized the best of what the program was trying to accomplish with all of its patients.

I explained that if the randomization process picked the code number assigned to Harold then he would be interviewed in my study; otherwise, not. As it turned out Harold's number came up and I was to conduct the interview with him. We arranged to have the interview at a nearby diner since Harold worked near my home and it was impossible for him to have a quiet and confidential talk at his busy office. He was most eager to be interviewed.

Harold, of course, had graduated from MCDC. He was in the program for approximately two and a half years. He went through reentry status and was later deemed to have successfully completed treatment.

Given what was said about him, I was particularly eager to conduct this interview. The interview confirmed many of the impressions that former therapists and counselors had of him. Harold was well dressed and athletic looking. Tall, with dark complexion, trim, he was talkative, yet introspective. He was a proud young man of twenty-six years old. He was very keen about reestablishing contacts with any of his former co-patients and was hoping that I might be able to assist him in this endeavor. Of course, I was unable to offer him that kind of help, so I suggested he approach the professional staff at Manhasset.

The interview established that he was a light drinker of alcoholic beverages and did not use any other drugs. He had an older sister who was still heavily involved in psychedelic drug use who he carefully avoided.

Although he was married and had his own home, he maintained very close ties to his family. He worked in his father's business as an office manager where he did anything from low level deliveries of computer parts to high level managerial work in hiring and firing professional employees. He made a salary in the $50,000 range.

His wife was several years older than he, and she was employed as a school administrator. They had no children, but were planning to start raising a family in the next few years. True to staff expectations, Harold and his wife lived in a large house in an expensive subdivision of the wealthy community of Great Neck.

Harold felt much gratitude for the Manhasset program and the direction it gave him when he was—as he saw it—a lost, angry, and foolish adolescent. He said he liked to go back to the treatment center periodically to find out what had happened to some of his old friends. He also enjoyed going to some of the center's social events, and regretted that there was not more post-treatment contact among former patients.

Harold reported no post-treatment criminal involvements. He also showed no current psychological symptoms, although he indicated some minor psychiatric troubles in the post-treatment time period. Since leaving the program he had finished two years of college. He said that someday soon he hopes to return to college to 'catch up with' his wife. Right now, however, business commitments were so pressing that school—even on a limited basis—was out of the question.

Harold seemed to be a good representative of someone that had benefitted from treatment. One may wonder whether there were others like him that also succeeded in putting their lives in order, but who did so without participating in the day care drug treatment.

Although Harold Rosen was well known at MCDC, few people remembered Alex Templeton. Alex remained a patient for approximately five months, so perhaps his short tenure may help account for the fact that few staff members remembered him. The director, however, remembered Alex as the patient with the famous parents.

Alex's stepfather was a nationally known figure, a very prolific professional writer and expert on the state of the arts and humanities who was frequently called upon to serve on presidential commissions and render expert testimony at congressional hearings. Alex's mother was not undistinguished either; she was a well-known fashion designer; her opinions and ideas on women's fashion often appear in women's apparel magazines.

When Alex came into day care, he presented little to distinguish himself except his notoriety. He had a long history of mental health treatments in a variety of settings. He also could boast about an imposing list of schools attended—at various private, public, and boarding institutions. At the intake, the psychiatrist was also struck by Alex's effeminate behavior, and remarked in the evaluation report that here was a young man with obvious sexual identification problems. One of the interesting things Alex did at the intake interview was make a list of the many drugs he had consumed. Alex's list nearly filled half a page of legal tablet size, enumerating some forty-four drugs. He had not missed many of the commonly and uncommonly used drugs and psychotropic medications in existence. This seemed rather remarkable considering his tender age of only sixteen years.

Shortly after the letter announcing the follow-up interviews went out I received a telephone call at my office from Alex's stepfather. He informed me that Alex had died about two years earlier, having committed suicide while under the influence of alcohol and cocaine. At the time, his stepson had been living in San Diego, California, in an inexpensive rooming house. He hung himself with his pants belt from a water pipe in the dingy basement apartment he occupied. After he had left Manhasset, he had been through a succession of different psychiatric hospitals, saw an incalculable number of private psychotherapists and obviously had gotten worse.

Thus, the contrast in post-treatment adaptations between Harold Rosen and Alex Templeton could not be more diverging. Of course, when reviewing individual cases, an endless array of potential explanations present themselves. Yet, one wonders what might have happened to Alex if he had completed the course of treatment at Manhasset and if he would still be alive today.

Of all the questions raised about Manhasset's program one of the most important is if its treatment effectively encourages the relinquishment of drug abuse among its adolescent clientele. What happened to those completing the program years afterward? Were they likely to be any less drug involved than others with similar drug abuse problems who did not participate in the program? Did those remaining in treatment gain any other benefits in their overall social functioning compared with program dropouts? These were the questions that guided the development of this chapter.

As previously mentioned, in amassing the sample of respondents little difficulty was encountered in locating and gaining the cooperation of those former patients who spent a year or more in treatment. The analysis sample ultimately consisted of twenty such patients: fifteen that graduated from the program and five others that spent at least a year in treatment. More resistance was encountered among those who had been short-term patients. There was a decidedly greater reluctance to participate among short term patients; only 72% (twenty-eight persons) agreed to be interviewed, while 87% of longer-term patients expressed a similar willingness to cooperate.

Moreover, Manhasset short-stay patients did not fit into a neat category of remaining untreated. Of the twenty-eight former patients staying less than six months in treatment at Manhasset nearly half—thirteen respondents—spent an average of forty-two months receiving care in a variety of other mental health and drug treatment facilities. Considering their extensive additional drug and psychiatric treatments, these thirteen former patients were excluded from most of this analysis. Consequently, this chapter compares twenty long-stay MCDC patients with another fifteen former patients, all of whom withdrew from the Manhasset program within six months, and all had received less than a year of treatment elsewhere since leaving Manhasset. Eighty percent of the minimally treated group had received less than a total of six months of treatment elsewhere since leaving the day care program. At the time of the follow-up, anywhere from three to eight years had elapsed since these patients had last completed/or withdrew from the Manhasset program.

I first examined the issue of whether treated respondents (those remaining at the program for at least a year) differed from program dropouts (those staying less than six months) in the pattern of their use of alcohol and drugs prior to entering treatment at Manhasset. Drug abuse patterns at intake for both groups were somewhat similar, but long-stay patients were somewhat less drug involved at intake compared to their counterparts who withdrew. There were no differences noted in the types of drugs consumed by both populations, but short-stay patients reported higher levels of drug use. Sixty percent of withdrawing patients used their chiefly abused drug at least twice or three times daily. By contrast, only a quarter of long-term patients reported such high levels of abuse. This difference was statistically significant ($p < .001$). In other respects, however, drug use patterns among the two groups were similar. Both groups reported abusing the same number and types of drugs and disclosed similar patterns in the frequency of subsidiary drug abuse.

At follow-up the patterns of drug abuse among the two groups were noticeably different. Marijuana, one of the chiefly abused drugs at intake, still remained the most widely used illegal drug. Nearly half of all these respondents (47%) reported occasional to frequent marijuana use at follow-up. Differences were striking among those remaining in and withdrawing from treatment: only 20% of long-term patients reported using marijuana at least several times a week, but two-thirds of program dropouts reported such levels of marijuana use ($p < .05$).

Follow-up differences in cocaine use between the two groups showed the same pattern. Only 20% of long-stay patients reported using cocaine, compared to 60% of short-stay patients. This was significant with Chi Square at the .01 level. Barbiturate use among the two groups also varied. Ten percent of patients spending a year or more at Manhasset reported using barbiturates, compared with 20% among their short-stay counterparts, but this difference failed to achieve statistical significance.

Alcohol consumption also varied among those taking and leaving drug treatment. Respondents were asked how frequently on a weekly basis they drank alcoholic beverages; they also provided information on the numbers of

Table 4-1.
Time in Treatment by Drug Score

	DRUG SCORE					
	0	1	2	3	4	5
TIME IN TREATMENT						
Treated year or more	1	7	4	2	3	3
Treated less than 6 mos.	0	2	1	3	5	4
Totals	1	9	5	5	8	7

Kendall's Tau B = -.31   Significance = .02

drinks (and ounces of alcohol) usually consumed during drinking episodes. No discernible differences were noted between either group in the numbers drinking daily or several times weekly. Program dropouts, however, reported much greater consumption during drinking episodes: 60% reported usually taking six or more drinks when drinking; among those staying at Manhasset for at least a year the comparable figure was only 15%. This difference was significant with Chi Square at the .01 level.

An overall index of drug abuse was developed, combining alcohol and drug consumption. After carefully studying all the drug use response data the following scale was created to measure the increasing gradient of drug abuse: (0) = no use of drugs and no alcohol consumption; (1) = no use of drugs and moderate alcohol consumption; (2) = no use of drugs and high alcohol consumption; (3) = heavy use of marijuana and no hard drug use; (4) = one hard drug consumed; (5) = two or more hard drugs consumed.[1] The composite drug abuse scale was moderately correlated with duration of treatment. Those receiving treatment were concentrated toward the low end of the drug abuse scale; for program dropouts, contrastingly, responses tended to congregate at the higher end. See Table 4-1.

Other differences were observed in post-treatment adaptations of the two groups. Program dropouts were more likely to have had problems with the law since leaving Manhasset, compared with longer-term patients. Among those who withdrew prematurely from treatment only one had never been arrested (7%) and 53% had been arrested on two or more occasions. Among those remaining in treatment 55% had never been arrested and 25% were arrested twice or more (p < .01). Program dropouts were also more likely to have spent time in jail. Forty-six percent had been in jail for at least two months since leaving treatment, contrasted with 5% among longer term patients (p < .001).

The driver license records of both groups of respondents were also investigated. More long-term patients had driver's licenses compared to program dropouts, 90% as compared to 67%. Among the licensed drivers the numbers of citations, infractions, accidents, and injuries reported by both groups was largely similar.

Yet, when I examined drug-related driving offenses the results suggested the possibility of a trend with short-term patients having more of such arrests. Thirty percent of short-term patients had one or more drunk driving arrests, as compared to 6% among the long-term patients. This difference approached but fell short of statistical significance ($p = .12$).

Another dimension of post-treatment functioning concerned the educational attainment of respondents. Former patients were asked how many years of full-time schooling they had completed since they left treatment. They were also asked about their overall educational attainment. Considering that most respondents were in their middle twenties at the time of follow-up (90% were twenty-one or over) and from middle to upper social status origins (nearly half—48%—had fathers working in managerial, professional, or proprietor occupations) it was somewhat surprising to note that very few had obtained four-year college degrees. In our entire sample of forty-eight, only two had completed such a degree. The data suggest that teenage drug abuse sharply reduces the scholastic attainments of those affected. One-third of all our respondents never completed high school, 58% finished high school or had obtained their G.E.D. equivalencies, and only 9% had undertaken some college course work.

Trends in the predicted direction were noted in educational attainment by duration of treatment. Ninety percent of long-term patients, but only two-thirds of program dropouts, had any further education after leaving Manhasset; 75% of long-term patients, compared to less than half of dropouts, completed two or more years of school since they had been in day care. The probabilities of both of these trends fell slightly short of the .05 level of significance.

Among the program dropout population almost half (47%) had not completed high school, 43% had finished high school or an equivalency, and 7% had done some college work. For the patients remaining in treatment longer the comparable figures were 15%, 70% and 15% respectively ($p < .01$).

Occupational accomplishments also varied between these two groups. While both groups displayed a similar likelihood of having work, the data showed more longer-term patients holding higher status jobs where they had a greater chance of gaining higher earnings.

Dropouts and long term patients alike reported that approximately three-fourths of both groups had been regularly employed during the last twelve months. Chronic unemployment (being out of work nine to twelve months during the last year) was reported for only a small fraction of respondents: 7% of dropouts and 10% among long-term patients. Yet, more short-term patients

Table 4-2.
Duration of Treatment by Number of Psychological Problems

	NUMBER OF PSYCHOLOGICAL PROBLEMS		
	0	1	2 or more
	percent (frequency)		
DURATION OF TREATMENT			
Short-stay	36 (5)	7 (1)	57 (8)
Long-stay	65 (13)	10 (2)	25 (5)
Totals	(18)	(3)	(13)

```
Chi Square= 3.63559 with 2 degrees of freedom
Significance= .1624
Pearson's R= -.32044 Significance= .0323
```

reported being out of work from one to six months: 27% as compared to 10%, although none of these differences were statistically significant.

The most apparent trend in work differences between the two groups was in the status of the positions they held. Greater numbers of long-term patients held managerial or white-collar occupations, 35% as compared to 7%. More short-term patients held semi- and unskilled manual jobs, 33% as compared to 15%, differences that came close to achieving statistical significance (p = .109).

Still another area of post-treatment adaptations explored was the psychological health of respondents. A summary list of questions pertaining to mental health functioning was included from the Addiction Severity Index (McLellan et al., 1980). Subjects were asked if during the previous month they had experienced any of the following problems: (a) serious depression, (b) serious anxiety or tension, (c) hallucinations, (d) trouble understanding, concentrating, or remembering, (e) trouble controlling violent behavior, (f) serious thoughts of suicide, or (g) attempted suicide. Table 4-2 gives evidence of a trend indicating more psychiatric symptoms reported by short-stay patients. Although the differences only approached significance with Chi Square, they did produce a significant correlation with Pearson's R.

Analysis of each of the separate items composing this psychological problems scale showed short-stay patients to be more likely to be experiencing serious anxiety and tension and having trouble in controlling violent inclinations. In the other respects, psychological profiles were much the same as those given by long-stay patients.

Still another behavioral area investigated was former patients' conventional social participation. A seven-point scale was developed indicating a person's level of social (and civic) affiliation; respondents were asked whether they possessed a driver's license, credit card, bank account, library card, voter registration status, and if they had attended religious services during the past year. Eighty-five percent of long-stay patients reported three or more of such conventional social affiliations as contrasted with 46% among the short-stay patients. The trend unmistakably showed reduced conventional civic involvements among program dropouts (p < .01).

A final aspect of social functioning concerned the family interaction patterns of the two groups of respondents. In many respects family behavior patterns among these groups of respondents were not substantially different. Somewhat more of the withdrawing patients were currently living with their parents at the time of the interview and reported less than harmonious relationships with their mothers than was true of long-stay patients, but the differences were considerably short of statistical significance. However, both sets of respondents indicated similar proportions having positive relationships with their fathers and siblings.

Statistically significant differences were noted regarding living with a girlfriend. Forty percent of short-stay patients reported living with a girlfriend during the year prior to the interview which compared to only 10% among long-stay patients (p < .05). The marriage rate was comparable in both groups; 27% of program dropouts were married, versus 35% among the long-term patients.

More of the program dropouts indicated they had parented children: 27% reported becoming parents, whereas none of the long-stay patients had done so. These differences were significant at the .01 level. When one considers that the long-stay patients were generally older than the program dropouts these patterns become all the more impressive.

Thus, in summing up the differences between the short- and long-stay patients a great many divergences between the two groups are apparent. Long-stay patients were using less drugs and alcohol after treatment; they were less likely to have been arrested and jailed. They had fewer drunk-driving charges levied against them, although the differences fell short of statistical significance. They had completed more formal schooling and tended to hold higher status jobs. They also reported fewer psychological problems and showed higher levels of civic and social participation.

Those who spurned drug treatment continued, on the average, to use more drugs. They had higher arrest rates and more psychological difficulties. While their labor force participation was comparable to the treated group, more worked at lower status jobs and were living in consensual unions.

What accounts for these differences? Was it produced as a result of the treatment experiences that some received? Could it be related to the greater drug use characterizing dropout patients when they first began treatment? Another possible explanation could be the social differences linked with those withdrawing from and completing care. As the preceding analysis in chapter

3 demonstrated, those presenting themselves for drug treatment were by no means a homogeneous group. Patients varied greatly from one another and these differences were associated with variations in treatment participation. Since differences in age, parental social status, and other factors affected treatment participation and completion, they would also be expected to be linked with post-treatment adaptations.

But it was first necessary to establish whether this follow-up sample of former day center patients exhibited comparable patterns that were noted in the larger clinic files sample. Consistent with the findings in the larger random sample, short-stay patients tended to be younger at intake than long-stay patients. Sixty-four percent of the program dropouts were fifteen years of age or less at intake, as compared with only 29% among long-stay patients (p = .036).

Other differences tended to follow the patterns found in the larger random sample. Proportionately more long-stay patients came from upper status homes, were of Jewish background, and were less likely to have committed serious crimes prior to intake. More long-stay patients' fathers and mothers had mental health or drug treatments elsewhere prior to intake. None of the above differences were less than or equal to the .05% probability level, although some came close.

The only other striking difference noted was between those recognized as depressed at intake. Those described as depressed at intake predominated among short-term patients (78%), compared to only 20% among long-term patients, yielding a Chi Square value that was significant at the .001 level.

At this phase of the analysis I attempted to assess whether the differences in follow-up outcomes were caused by program participation or whether they were the results of characteristics of patients at intake. For this analysis I decided to focus on the issue of post-treatment drug use. Inasmuch as the rehabilitative services were primarily focused on drug consumption this seemed like the most appropriate dependent variable to use. (The question of how post-treatment drug use affected other areas of conduct such as criminality, work, psychological problems and other things will be investigated in the next chapter.)

Multiple regression was employed in an attempt to establish some sense of the relative contribution of each of the independent variables in explaining variations in the dependent variable. The dependent variable, drug score (DRGSCORE), consisted of a six-point scale already described. The regression equation included the following independent variables: (1) frequency of drug use at intake; (2) father's occupational rank; (3) if either parent had a history of drug abuse; (4) patient's criminal record at intake; (5) mental health care history of mother; (6) mental health care history of father; (7) religion (Jews versus non-Jews); (8) patient's depression at intake; (9) patient's age; (10) experience of treatment (a year or more versus less than six months); (11) age at first use of drugs.

Table 4-3.
Pearson Product-Moment Correlations with DRGSCORE: Initial Screening
of Zero-Order Correlation Coefficients

	r value	probability
1) frequency of drug use at intake	.09	.30
2) father's occupational rank	.19	.14
3) parental history of drug abuse	-.16	.19
4) patient's criminal record	.15	.20
5) mental health care history of mother	.05	.40
6) mental health care history of father	-.03	.43
7) religion	-.27	.06
8) patient's depression	.23	.09
9) patient's age	-.28	.05
10) day care treatment experience	-.36	.02
11) age at first use of drugs	-.46	.003

An initial run using all the independent variables yielded an R Square of .35 against the dependent variable. Zero-order correlation coefficients of each variable were noted and those yielding the least influential results were dropped from subsequent analyses. The coefficients of each of the eleven initially included variables are listed in table 4.3.

The results showed drug use at intake and the mental health treatment histories of parents to have a negligible association with the dependent variable. These variables were therefore dropped. Note here that age at first use of drugs and treatment experience were the most powerful predictors.

The next multiple regression with the eight remaining variables yielded an overall R Square of .33. A backward regression model was also applied which eliminated, one by one, each of the weaker variables from the regression equation (Norusis, 1986). The strongest variables remaining in the equation when all others were removed were treatment experience and age at first use. These variables together accounted for an R Square value of .28. All the other remaining variables only added a total of .05 to explaining the variations in drug scores. Thus, these two variables alone contributed nearly 90% of all the explained variance. Table 4-4 lists each of the variables that were present in the backward regression equation, their zero-order correlation coefficients, beta weights, and significance.

Table 4-4.
Zero-Order Correlation Coefficients and Beta Weights against DRGSCORE

	r value	Beta weight	Sig F
1) father's occupational rank	.19	-.05	.88
2) parental history of drug abuse	-.16	-.15	.47
3) patient's criminal record	.15	.09	.77
4) religion	-.27	-.21	.32
5) patient's depression	.23	-.05	.99
6) patient's age	-.28	.12	.85
7) day care treatment experience	-.36	-.30	.09
8) age at first use	-.46	-.41	.01

Thus, the evidence from the multiple regression—the size of correlation coefficients, beta weights, and R Square values—clearly indicates that treatment experience and age at first use were the most powerful variables that were established from this array of potential predictors. The other variables that were included here appear to have a more indirect association with the dependent variable. One might speculate that their connection to the dependent variable may lie in their association with treatment experience, which has already been established.

To add further confirmation to the above scheme the multiple regression analysis was applied to the entire interview sample of forty-eight cases. Each of the above variables were included in this analysis. Treatment experience, of course, was redefined in light of the present inclusion of the twenty-eight cases of former patients who had been treated in a variety of other mental health and drug treatment programs. A new variable was created to explore the significance of all treatment experiences, including day care and post-Manhasset treatment experiences. It consisted simply of the total number of months that former patients spent in treatment at various different mental health, drug rehabilitation, or self-help care facilities.

The R Square value of all eight independent variables against the dependent variable, DRGSCORE, was .21. Table 4-5 lists the values of each of the zero-order correlation coefficients, beta weights, F values, and significance.

Reviewing the correlation coefficients it is clear that the number of months in treatment and age at first use were much higher than any of the other variables in accounting for variations in drug scores. When all of the other six variables except treatment experiences and age at first use were removed from the regression equation the R Square decreased modestly to .16. This analysis has confirmed the earlier one, documenting the important role of treatment ex-

Table 4-5.
Zero-Order Correlation Coefficients, Beta Weights, F Values and
Significance

	Zero-order r	Beta weight	F value	Sig F
1) father's occupational rank	.03	-.11	.380	.54
2) parental hist. of drug abuse	-.11	-.15	.888	.35
3) patient's criminal record	.11	.04	.003	.95
4) religion	.02	-.06	.122	.72
5) patient's depression	.15	.12	.594	.44
6) patient's age	-.11	.17	.789	.38
7) treatment experiences	-.34	-.37	5.501	.02
8) age at first use	-.26	-.26	2.291	.14

periences and age at first use in affecting variations in post-treatment drug consumption and abuse.

In examining Table 4-5 one can discern the relative importance of treatment experiences, over age at first use, in accounting for variations in drug abuse scores. Of all the variables considered here, treatment experiences was the only one to achieve statistical significance. It yielded the highest zero-order correlation coefficient and beta weight. It alone accounted for more than half of all the explained variation offered by all the variables combined (R Square = .12). Age at first use alone accounted for an increment of .04 to R Square when it was added to the multiple regression equation.

In an effort to further illuminate the relative contributions of each of the predictor variables against the dependent variable, DRGSCORE, stepwise and forward selection regression models were also computed for the data. While the amount of explained variance changed in some instances, the relative values of predictor variables compared to each other remained as shown in the backward regression model. Given the large number of predictor variables and the small number of cases for analysis readers are advised to accept these multiple regression findings tentatively.

Summing up this evidence from the follow-up of former patients three to eight years after treatment, the data suggested that day care helped reduce drug abuse. Those who spent at least a year or more in care were much less drug involved than those who withdrew from treatment within six months. Those who were under care longer were much less inclined to be using marijuana and cocaine at follow-up. While long-term patients drank alcohol about as often as dropouts they tended to drink far more moderately. The longer-treated group also appeared to be less likely to engage in subsequent criminal activity. They tended to get more schooling and held higher status jobs compared to dropouts. They also reported fewer psychological difficulties and gave more evidence of conventional social participation.

Multiple regression provided additional support to substantiate the importance of treatment experience and day care over most all of the sociodemographic factors in explaining continuing drug abuse. How old youngsters were when they entered treatment and at follow-up, their history of depression, religious backgrounds, parents' social status, drug abuse history, and mental health treatment histories made less substantial and insignificant contributions in accounting for variation in patterns of post-treatment drug abuse. The only pretreatment factor to show any importance in determining continuing drug abuse was the timing of when adolescents started using drugs. Those starting to use drugs at younger ages were more likely to resist taking treatment and less likely to remain drug-free years later.

The evidence offers some preliminary support for the utility of day care in treating adolescent multidrug abuse. Day care programs like Manhasset's obviously represent a less costly alternative than residential treatments which also must provide room and board to clients and round the clock professional supervision. Future researchers will find it advantageous to investigate what the actual savings would amount to in running day care versus residential treatment programs.

Of course, there are many adolescent drug abuse clients whose parental resources are so meager and where interference from drug-using peers is such a compelling force that only by removal from their familiar surroundings is it possible to achieve any significant rehabilitative results. However, this evidence would appear to support efforts toward expanding the availability of day care, since by offering day care more widely it should be possible to stretch resources earmarked for treatment further to serving a larger base of adolescent clientele.

Note

1. In the drug abuse scale high alcohol consumption was defined by drinking four or more drinks during drinking episodes. Heavy marijuana use was regarded as using the drug several times weekly or more frequently. Additional analyses with this scale will be found in the next chapter.

5

Correlates of Continuing Drug Abuse

In this chapter I identify some additional behavioral patterns linked to different levels of post-treatment drug use. It has been well established by prior studies that teenage drug abusers are destined to encounter a variety of problems during their adult lives (Newcomb and Bentler, 1988). They are more inclined to engage in criminal conduct, to have trouble getting and keeping jobs, completing school, and in achieving upward social mobility (Kleinman, Wish, Deren, and Rainone, 1986; Johnson et al., 1986; Jessor, Chase, and Donovan, 1980; Johnston, 1974; Glickman and Utada, 1983; Newcomb and Bentler, 1988). They are also more prone to a variety of psychological difficulties, increased suicide, and depression, among other problems (Gove, Geerkin, and Hughes, 1979; Paton, Kessler, and Kandel, 1977; Mellinger et al., 1975; Newcomb and Bentler, 1988). Social marginality is another concomitant of high drug consumption; those so inclined tend to have more disrupted and conflicted relationships with their families and with society at large (Smith and Fogg, 1975; Glickman and Utada, 1983). It was suspected that the Manhasset data would confirm such patterns. The purpose here was to extend earlier findings and probe whether there may be some important concomitants to post-treatment drug use that had not been already recognized.

Secondly, an additional aim was to gauge the consequences linked with varying degrees of post-treatment drug use. I wanted to investigate what levels of post-treatment drug consumption would be likely to inspire adult adjustment problems. Also, I wondered whether it was necessary for former drug abusers to remain abstinent to avoid adjustment problems; it seemed plausible, but by no means certain, that nonproblematical behavior patterns could be sustained with low levels of post-treatment drug consumption.

Lastly, a further goal of this chapter was to evaluate the value of day care treatment for young adults. With the cohort of Manhasset patients as a guidepoint, I wanted to gauge how many young adult former patients were likely to be improved from treatment; how many unimproved; and what the commonmost kinds of post-treatment adaptations of former patients were. These questions guided the present analysis.

Characteristics of the Follow-Up Population

As mentioned earlier, all these respondents were white, non-Hispanic males. Most were young: at the time of follow-up a large majority (86%) were between twenty and twenty-five. The mean was 22.5 years of age. Despite their young age, most had accumulated years of experience with drugs. On average they had started drug use 9.5 years prior to this follow-up; and seven to eight years had elapsed since they began a regular pattern of drug use.

Similarly, a long period had passed since they first entered treatment at Manhasset. The mean follow-up for our respondents occurred 6.8 years after admission; the shortest follow-up cases (6%) were interviewed four years after entry.

Drug Use Patterns

I anticipated that the data would show a close convergence between the following elements: (1) the frequency of drug use; (2) the number of drugs taken and their illegal standing; and (3) the subjective awareness of problems inherent in such action. If such an interrelated pattern was evident, then this would a good indication of the utility of the scale of drug use (presented in the last chapter) as depicting movement along a continuum to higher degrees of abuse.

In the last chapter I discussed the measure of drug abuse, consisting of a six-point scale with the following points: (0) = no use of drugs and no alcohol consumption; (1) = no use of drugs and moderate alcohol consumption; (2) = no use of drugs and high alcohol consumption; (3) = heavy use of marijuana and no hard drug use; (4) = one hard drug consumed; (5) = two or more hard drugs consumed. The following breakdown of use patterns was noted for our forty-eight respondents at follow-up.

Readers should note that of the five individuals scoring zero on the drug score scale in the table above, three were in fact patients in drug-free residential treatment settings at the time of interview. As the following analysis will show, most of the currently drug-free respondents had long histories of heavy past drug use. Consequently, on a number of the problem dimensions surveyed curvilinear patterns were noted showing the hard drug users and the presently abstinent with the highest values, compared to all other drug-using groups.

Looking across the scale it is noted that alcohol consumption generally rises as one goes from the low to the high end of the drug score scale. Although the pattern was not completely linear, the percent taking six or more drinks during drinking episodes rose from a low of 0% to a high of 67%. Among hard drug users taking two or more such drugs, drinking still remained heavy with over half usually taking six or more drinks whenever they drank alcoholic beverages. Marijuana use also remained significant among each of the higher abusing drug groups. Forty-four and 78% of persons in each of the two hard drug groups still reported using marijuana several times a week. The frequency of

Table 5-1.
Drinking and Marijuana Consumption by Drug Scale Score

	None	Low Alc	Hi Alc	Mari-juana	One hard	Two hard
DRGSCORE VALUES	(0)	(1)	(2)	(3)	(4)	(5)
Percent (Number)	10(5)	25(12)	15(7)	13(6)	19(9)	19(9)
Percent having 6 or more drinks when drinking	0	0	42	33	67	56
Percent using marijuana several times weekly or more	0	0	0	100	44	78

marijuana use was strongly correlated with the use of other drugs. Table 5-2 shows how marijuana use increased among each abuse category.

Most subjects either did not use marijuana at all (twenty-nine) or used it at least weekly (seventeen). Eight subjects reported using marijuana several times a week, and nine reported daily or greater use. Second, all six of the subjects who used marijuana but not hard drugs reported high marijuana use patterns; all used the drug at least several times weekly. Heavy marijuana users who did not take hard drugs also tended to be heavy drinkers. All but one (a daily marijuana user) drank four or more drinks when drinking.

Those using one hard drug reported relatively modest abuse patterns of that drug. Only one (11%) indicated using his drug (usually cocaine) as frequently as several times weekly. Yet, we must acknowledge that this subgroup were inclined to rather high levels of marijuana and alcohol consumption. Two-

Table 5-2.
Marijuana Use by Drug Scale Score

	Used no other drugs	Used alcohol, no hard drugs	One hard drug	Two or more hard drugs
Percent not using mari-juana	100	76	44	11
Percent using marijuana daily	0	8	22	56

Table 5-3.
Mean Drug-Related Reported Problems by Drug Scale Score

	None	Low Alc	Hi Alc	Mari- juana	One hard	Two hard
DRGSCORE VALUES	(0)	(1)	(2)	(3)	(4)	(5)
Percent (Number)	10(5)	25(12)	15(7)	13(6)	19(9)	19(9)
Mean number of alcohol-related problems reported	0	.67	1.9	3.2	2.8	3.4
Mean number of other drug problems reported	0	0	0	.67	.8	5.2

thirds reported taking six or more drinks during drinking episodes. And close to half (44%) said they used marijuana at least several times weekly.

Those at the highest point of the scale—using two or more hard drugs—reported overall high levels of drug use. Seventy-eight percent reported using one or more drugs at least several times weekly. While this group had somewhat lower alcohol consumption than the last mentioned category, their use of marijuana was considerable. More than three-fourths claimed to use marijuana at least several times weekly.

All subjects were asked if any of the drugs they consumed ever caused them any trouble in relation to work or school, family and friendship relations, health, the law or finances. Respondents were also asked four separate questions in relation to alcohol consumption: whether they had experienced blackouts, hangovers, stomach distress, and extended drunks during the last year. A correspondence was noted between scale points and the recognition of drug problems. Table 5-3 shows how each higher drug use scale point led to a greater recognition of drug-related difficulties. Those in the highest use category, apparently, had a substantially elevated level of awareness of drug-related problems.

Thus, my initial hypothesis between the frequency of drug use, the number of drugs taken and the recognition of drug-related problems seemed to be supported. The data suggest a steep rise in the perception of drug-related problems when individuals consume at least two hard drugs.

Criminal Involvements

Consistent with previous research findings there was a close correspondence between the degree of drug abuse and the criminal activities of former pa-

Table 5-4.
Drug Abuse and Self-Reported Crime in Prior Two Months

	None	Low Alc	Hi Alc	Mari- juana	One hard	Two hard
DRGSCORE VALUES	(5)	(12)	(7)	(6)	(9)	(9)
		Percent/(Number)				
Had engaged in any of the listed crimes in last two months	0(0)	8(1)	17(1)	0(0)	33(3)	44(4)

tients. Respondents were asked if they had committed any of the following common criminal activities during the two month period preceding the interview: shoplifting, pickpocketing, burglary, robbery, forgery, auto theft, blackmail, arson, vandalism, assault, mugging, prostitution, drug dealing, etc. (See Appendix B for specific questions). Self-reported crime closely followed the degree of drug abuse, as shown in Table 5-4. (Kendall's Tau B was .27, significant at the .02 level.)

The data also showed a pattern linking drug abuse with the likelihood of spending more time in jail during the post-treatment period (see Table 5-5). Respondents were divided into three categories, those with: (1) no jail time; (2) less than a month of jail; and (3) more than a month in jail. Kendall's Tau B yielded a value of .26, where p < .01.

Respondents were also asked how many times they had been arrested for any crimes since they were in treatment. The results showed a nonlinear pattern. As expected, moving across the scale to higher abuse levels there was a trend toward a rising number of post-treatment arrests. Yet, the highest post-treatment arrest rates were reported by those not using any drugs and alcohol

Table 5-5.
Drug Abuse and Time Spent in Jail since Treatment

	None	Low Alc	Hi Alc	Mari- juana	One hard	Two hard
DRGSCORE VALUES	(5)	(12)	(7)	(6)	(9)	(9)
		Percent/(Number)				
No jail time	20(1)	42(5)	57(4)	50(3)	0(0)	11(1)
Jail, less than a month	60(3)	42(5)	43(3)	17(1)	78(7)	33(3)
Jail, more than a month	20(1)	17(2)	0(0)	33(2)	22(2)	56(5)

Table 5-6.
Arrest History since Treatment

	None	Low Alc	Hi Alc	Mari- juana	One hard	Two hard
DRGSCORE VALUES	(5)	(12)	(7)	(6)	(9)	(9)
		Percent/(Number)				
Mean No. post-treatment arrests	2.60	1.0	.71	.67	1.89	2.33

at all. The data revealed that some of the presently abstinent members of the sample had earlier post-treatment periods when they had engaged in high drug consumption. Of these five cases where respondents reported no drug use during the two month period preceding the interview, three respondents indicated three or more post-treatment arrests. In each of these cases the subject indicated that he had had an extended period of high drug consumption in the intervening years since being at Manhasset. Two of the three high crime-involved respondents were current patients of drug rehabilitation programs at the time of the interview. The other was currently being maintained on an antidepressant medication.

As a final part to this survey of criminal activities I examined the driving license records of respondents. Here comparisons were confined to all respondents possessing current drivers' licenses. No differences were noted between those at the high end of the drug score scale and those at the low end with respect to their overall numbers of driving infractions. Yet, a trend seemed apparent in the numbers charged with drug-related driving offenses. Only 6% (one of eighteen) of those at the low end of the drug score scale but 22% (four out of eighteen) of those at the high end of the scale had any drunk driving charges. However, given the small number of cases for these comparisons, Chi Square values failed to reach significance (p = .14).

In summary, it was only among hard drug users (and former hard drug users) that criminal activities were frequently reported.

Work and Schooling Patterns

Another area of inquiry considered the linkages between post-treatment drug use and work or educational involvements. I already mentioned the apparent downward mobility of our sample of former drug abuse patients. Despite the fact that nearly half (48%) of their fathers and a quarter of their mothers had taken four or more years of college, only two former patients (5%) had completed equivalent amounts of education at follow-up. Although 48% of fathers held managerial, professional, or proprietary occupations, only 8% of

Table 5-7.
Drug Abuse, Unemployment and Current School Participation

	None	Low Alc	Hi Alc	Mari-juana	One hard	Two hard
DRGSCORE VALUES	(5)	(12)	(7)	(6)	(9)	(9)
		Percent/(Number)				
Percent un-employed 3 or more months in last year	20(1)	16(2)	28(2)	33(2)	0(0)	66(6)
Percent going to school full or part time last year	40(2)	42(5)	28(2)	17(1)	11(1)	0(0)

their sons were similarly employed. Of course, many of these young men had yet to reach their peaks of occupational and educational attainments.

The positions held by these respondents were many and varied. They included the following occupations: salesman, truckdriver, construction laborer, carpenter, telephone solicitor, office manager, printer, chef, short order cook, office manager, floor waxer, landscaper, refrigeration mechanic, auto mechanic, plumbing contractor, dispatcher, security guard, stockroom attendant, production manager, machine operator, school custodian, baker, clerk, and pressman, among others. Among those few holding managerial or high-paying positions most were employed in family-owned businesses (three out of four such cases). The absence of professional employment among respondents is striking, for although professional occupations are relatively common in Nassau County and among the respondents' parents, none of those sampled were reported to be teachers, lawyers, accountants, engineers, etc.

Most respondents were, however, employed at the time of the interview and throughout the year preceding the interview. Nearly two-thirds (62%) reported working or going to school at least forty or more weeks during the previous year.

Seven respondents (15%) reported being unemployed during most of the year prior to the interview. There was a correspondence between the drug abuse scale score and the likelihood of being unemployed. Table 5-7 shows how those at the highest point of the drug scale were more often unemployed than all others. Cross-tabulating drug abuse score with unemployment produced a Kendall's Tau B of .24, significant at the .03 level.

Present scholastic status was similarly linked with drug scale score. (Kendall's Tau B showed a correlation of .-32, where $p < .005$.) Almost none of those at the high end of the drug abuse scale were students during the previous year. Surprisingly, however, no differences were found between any of the drug

Table 5-8.
Drug Abuse and Current Work/School Involvements

	None	Low Alc	Hi Alc	Mari- juana	One hard	Two hard
DRGSCORE VALUES (5)	(12)	(7)	(6)	(9)	(9)	
Median weeks worked or went to school in last year	22	52	45	46	50	25
Percent working or going to school 40 or more weeks	40	75	71	67	89	22

using groups and overall educational attainment. No differences were noted between any of the groups in total years of school completed and/or years completed since release from Manhasset. Because of the relative youth of the sample, probably a longer term follow-up would be needed to fully assess the impact of drug involvement upon educational attainments.

One can think of steady employment and enrollment in an educational program as two indicators of degree of involvement in mainstream institutions. Therefore, I cross-tabulated the extent of work or education with drug use. A nonlinear pattern emerged. Both high drug abusers and abstainers were found to be the least likely to be steadily employed among all drug using subgroups. Using working or going to school forty or more weeks and the median number of weeks respondents worked (or went to school) showed great similarity. Table 5-8 displays the data.

By now it is probably clear why those at the high end of the drug abuse scale would be less steadily involved in work or school participation. On the other hand, it seemed unclear why those using no drugs at all would also tend to be irregularly employed. I suspected this had a great deal to do with the current patient status of respondents. For those who were current patients—either in residence at therapeutic communities, or in psychiatric hospitals, or in some other form of closely supervised therapy (e.g. day care or a group home)—such involvements would effectively reduce the use of recreational drugs. Similarly, treatment participation would effectively curtail availability for work or school. For the five respondents that were current patients of drug rehabilitation or psychiatric facilities all reported working minimally during the previous year. None of the five worked (or went to school) more than a total of thirty-two weeks. Drug scale scores of these five were concentrated at the low end of the scale; four of the five reported drug scale scores of one or less; and none took any illegal drugs.

Other work-related variables I examined in relation to drug use were occupational rank and earnings. The data presented in Table 5-9 supported this

Table 5-9.
Drug Abuse, Occupational Rank and Earnings

	None	Low Alc	Hi Alc	Mari- juana	One hard	Two hard
DRGSCORE VALUES	(5)	(12)	(7)	(6)	(9)	(9)
			Percent/(Number)			
Percent employed in non-manual occupations	18(2)	46(5)	9(1)	18(2)	0(0)	9(1)
Percent employed in manual job or unemployed	8(3)	19(7)	16(6)	11(4)	23(9)	22(8)
Percent earning over $20,000 in last year	6(1)	50(8)	0(0)	19(3)	25(4)	0(0)
Percent earning less than $20,000	13(4)	13(4)	22(7)	10(3)	16(5)	26(8)

hypothesis. Seventy-three percent of all of those engaged in nonmanual occupations were concentrated in the low drug use categories. Only three illegal drug users (27%) had attained a nonmanual occupation. Kendall's Tau B yielded a coefficient of -.28, which was significant at the .02 level.

The pattern with earnings was generally consistent. Over half (56%) of the higher earners were concentrated in the two lowest use categories. A sizable minority of those using marijuana and/or one hard drug still managed to maintain higher levels of earnings. Yet, among those using two or more hard drugs and high alcohol consumers there appeared to be a trend toward depressed earnings. Kendall's Tau B yielded a .20, where p < .06.

Psychological Problems

The Addiction Severity Index (McLellan et al., 1980) included questions pertaining to individual mental health functioning. Subjects were asked if during the previous month they had experienced any of the following problems: (a) serious depression, (b) serious anxiety or tension, (c) hallucinations, (c) trouble understanding, concentrating, or remembering, (e) trouble controlling violent behavior, (f) serious thoughts of suicide, or (g) attempted suicide. The results showed a very clear linear trend (see Table 5-10). The psychological problems scale yielded a Kendall's Tau B of .33, where p < .005. Analysis of the separate items of the scale showed four items to be particularly likely to increase with rising levels of drug abuse: serious depression, serious anxiety and tension, hallucinations, and violent inclinations.

Table 5-10.
Drug Abuse and Psychological Problems

	None	Low Alc	Hi Alc	Mari- juana	One hard	Two hard
DRGSCORE VALUES	(5)	(12)	(7)	(6)	(9)	(8)
		Percent/(Number)				
Percent reporting one or no psychological problems	80(4)	92(11)	60(5)	67(4)	55(5)	38(3)
Percent reporting two or more psychological problems	20(1)	8(1)	40(2)	33(2)	45(4)	52(5)

Family Living Trends

One of the surprising revelations of the research was a positive correlation between living with parents and drug abuse. Table 5-11 shows that a high proportion of heavy drug users were still living at their parent's home. Kendall's Tau B yielded a value of .42, which was significant well beyond the .001 level.

Consistent with earlier research findings, I had expected that those abusing drugs would be more inclined to be living with a partner outside of marriage, living alone, or with friends (others also engaged in high drug use). For example, Denise Kandel (1984) found that adult marijuana users were more likely to be living with a partner rather than in a formal marriage and less attached to conventional institutions. Among the nine respondents in the sample that lived with a girlfriend during the previous year, six had drug scale scores

Table 5-11.
Drug Abuse and Living with Parents

	None	Low Alc	Hi Alc	Mari- juana	One hard	Two hard
DRGSCORE VALUES	(5)	(12)	(7)	(6)	(9)	(9)
		Percent/(Number)				
Percent living with parents during last year	20(1)	8(1)	43(3)	33(2)	56(5)	78(7)

that were at the high end of the scale. This was consistent with Kandel's findings. However, when living with friends and alone were cross-tabulated with drug abuse scale scores no differences between high and low drug users were noted. No previous studies have found trends showing high proportions of heavy users to be living with parents.

Living with parents did not necessarily mean respondents lived only in their parental households throughout the year preceding the interview. In some cases this was true. In others, respondents lived in a variety of places: with parents, friends, by themselves, and at other times elsewhere. The pattern of having a variety of residences was common among many heavy drug users. Subjects were asked where they had lived most of the time during the previous year. Living with parents meant that a respondent had spent more time during the last year in that type of living arrangement than in any other. Those indicating that they had not lived with parents spent less time living in parental homes, and did not consider their parental homes as their primary residences for the last year.

These findings suggest several possible interpretations. All or some of these explanations may be correct and relevant. For one, young adult male drug abusers living with parents saved much money on living expenses, expanding their opportunities to buy drugs. Considering that many in the highest drug use category were irregularly employed and usually working in lower paying jobs, the saving created by living with parents would be greater under these circumstances.

For another, in a society priding economic independence and personal autonomy, to be an adult that lives with one's parents represents a discreditable position. It could contribute to a poorer sense of self-esteem, increased feelings of personal failure and depression, as one may be dependent upon the largess of one's parents and unable to support oneself. In the intimate environment of the family such individuals could be subjected to occasional ridicule on account of their apparent shortcomings—no good job, no school participation, bad company, etc. While roommates and others might be reluctant to offer criticism of such personal shortcomings, family members usually feel free to offer sometimes painful advice and judgments. I investigated whether those at the high end of the drug score scale reported any more strained relations with their parents. The results showed that similar proportions of both low and high drug abusers reported having conflicts with parents. Yet, when I compared those living with parents and those in all other living arrangements, the data showed more conflict-relations among those living at their parents' home. Sixty-three percent of those living at home reported negative, indifferent, or mixed relations with at least one parent, compared to 41% among those living independently of their parental homes. The differences yielded a Chi Square value of 2.17, which approached significance (p = .14). Evidently, the association between living at one's parental home and having conflict is strong enough to be noticed but not so strongly correlated in this small sample as to be seen across the different drug using groups.

Another possibility is a pattern of parental enabling. Enabling is a concept in the alcoholism treatment literature frequently used by therapeutic practitioners and members of Alcoholics Anonymous (Brown, 1985; Bepko, 1985). 'Enablers' or 'co-alcoholics' as they are sometimes called, typically assume an overprotective, overresponsible role in managing the life of the drug abuser. Consequently, it is argued, they make it easier for the substance abusers to pursue their drug-taking inclinations. I found few parents so inclined to support their child's pattern of drug abuse as to actually furnish them with drugs. Only 16% (seven cases) of all respondents had ever received any drugs from their parents. And of those, less than half were cases where parents had knowingly offered any drugs to their child. Parental provision of drugs was rare, and limited to a few isolated instances.

Yet, if enabling is important in accounting for these young adults' persisting drug abuse, I would speculate that parental support and encouragement of abuse would be more commonly manifested in other ways. Most often parents would not be willing to confront their child on their heavy drug use. Parents would be inclined to deny their child's use was all that heavy. They would be reluctant to set limits, or to eject their child from the house if they could not reduce or stop their use of drugs.

The data suggested enabling as a potential explanation. In one case a respondent's mother indicated to me that her son had been living with her and her husband during a period when he was engaged in heavy use of cocaine, psychedelic drugs, heroin, and alcohol and had also been implicated in a number of minor crimes in the neighborhood (barroom brawls, vagrancy, and petty thefts). After recognizing her disapproval of his conduct, I asked why she had not kicked him out of the house. She indicated that he would only go to live with his sister if that happened, and then he might do much worse. She viewed her daughter as having a corrupting influence on her son. At the time of the interview her son's whereabouts were unknown. He was hiding out from the law because of serious criminal charges and his parents were currently providing sanctuary to his wife and infant child.

In one other case, a respondent's appearance gave ready confirmation to his later admission of high drug use. The respondent spoke very slowly and answered questions after many long pauses. His eyes were reddened. There were many burn marks and scars all over his hands and forearms. (During the interview he later acknowledged heavy daily drinking, daily marijuana use, and greater than weekly use of cocaine and amphetamines.) Before meeting with him I was met at the door by his mother. She indicated to me that her son was still having a drug problem but it was not as bad as it had been in the past. She mentioned that she had tried to get him into treatment on several occasions, but that he had always resisted getting professional help. She added that treatment had not done much for her eldest son who has been in and out of drug rehabilitation centers and mental hospitals for years. She said she was glad that her son was willing to stay at home; this way she could help him avoid getting into trouble with the police and at least he ate regularly and had a roof over his head. If and when he should ever want to get treatment, she would be the first person to know about it and make sure that he got it.

These are vignettes rather than systematic data. I did not interview parents as a matter of course. However, they do suggest the plausibility of parental enabling as an explanation of why drug use was higher among respondents who lived in their parents' homes.

Parents may also have contributed to their sons' persistent drug abuse through a pattern of permissive socialization. All subjects were given an array of statements to respond to about the kinds the relationships they had with their parents when they were teenagers. Several items showed significant (or near significant) relationships to high drug abuse. These items clustered on a common theme of permissiveness. The statement, "my parents were very strict with me," showed fewer high drug users inclined to agree compared with low drug users. Nearly half (48%) of low drug users agreed on parental strictness, as compared to a third of high drug users. The statement, "parents set definite rules for controlling and deciding things you could do," also produced a parallel trend. Seventy-eight percent of low-abusing subjects agreed with this statement, compared to 41% of those among the high abuse categories. This was significant with Chi Square at the .01 level. More of the higher abusing subjects agreed with the statement that parents warned them not to do disapproved things again, but seldom punished them, 67% as compared to 39% among lower abusing subjects (p = .06 with Chi Square). Thus, the data showed a pattern of parental permissiveness among those at the high end of the drug abuse scale.

An alternative explanation for the higher abuse rates among those living with parents might be substance abuse among the parents, although this hypothesis was not supported by the data. Those at the high end of the drug abuse scale were no different from those at the low end on any of the indicators of parental substance abuse: whether fathers or mothers drank heavily during the last three years or ever before; whether parents ever used any illegal drugs (and the frequency of use); and whether Manhasset clinic records indicated any history of abuse of drugs when parents were initially screened. No trends were noted between any combination of these elements and the pattern of post-treatment drug abuse.

This finding goes against previous studies. Earlier studies found increased rates of alcoholism among the children of alcoholics (Cloninger et al. 1978; Goodwin, 1979; Goodwin et al., 1977). A study of opioid addicts found that those whose parents were alcoholics were more inclined to be concurrent alcoholics and to have more severe problems with alcohol abuse (Kosten, Rounsaville and Kleber, 1985). (However, that study did not establish that the pattern of opioid abuse itself differed in any way between those whose parents were and were not alcoholics.) Kandel found that parental use of hard liquor predicted adolescent use of hard liquor and other illicit drugs but not marijuana. Parental use of psychoactive drugs also predicted adolescent use of illicit drugs other than marijuana (Kandel, Kessler, and Margulies, 1978.) (In the case of marijuana use the peer group proved to have a far more decisive influence.)

Yet, while parental behavior in these studies has been shown to have had an impact in initiating early drug-taking, it remains to be established whether it also accounts for the persistence of polydrug abuse during adulthood. On the basis of the evidence collected here—among this sample of former day treatment drug clinic patients of white middle class males in their early twenties—the answer to explaining continuing high use will have to be found apart from parental imitation and modeling.

Still another possible explanation can be seen by also considering living with parents as a dependent variable. These young adults living with their parents may have been "losers" among their peers and in the larger community. Living with their parents could have been a refuge, a reflection that they were unable to carry on effective social relations. They may have been kicked out of houses and apartments, or had difficulty paying their bills. They may also have had problems in getting along with housemates. Most of the heavy drug users living with their parents also reported a diverse array of other living arrangements. Living with their parents may have represented a last resort choice and a sense of failing to succeed in society. Perhaps, with feelings of inadequacy, depression and the inclination to heavy drug use may have been encouraged.

To be sure, these findings linking parental residence and high drug abuse are most surprising and invite further speculation and research. Recent sociological writings have recognized possibilities for rising parent/child conflict with the fast growing pattern today of more young adults returning to live in their parental homes (Riche, 1987; Cowan, 1989; Schnaiberg and Goldenberg, 1989). Particularly among the middle classes, as contemporary economic conditions no longer permit many young adults to live in the affluent style they were accustomed to as children, many have sought to return to their parental homes, seeking to conserve their limited economic resources. Middle-aged parents, in turn, have begun to increasingly cherish their own independence and freedom, as many now enjoy unprecedented opportunities to pursue career and recreational interests. Many parents have grown comfortable in their so-called empty nests and resent new requests for support and assistance coming from their adult children. Now, an anomic situation often prevails in the parental households where all parties prize independence and autonomy and must cope with the daily realities of economic dependence. Drug abuse has rarely been discussed as one of the possible results from dealing with such issues, although our data suggests that it may become a more pervasive issue in the many families coping with this new problem of a 'crowded nest.' Further research will be needed to fully assess the significance of this correlation between persisting drug abuse and living arrangements where adult children remain as members of their parental households.

Table 5-12.
Drug Abuse and Having Many Close Friends Using Alcohol Heavily and One Illegal Drug or Two Illegal Drugs

	None	Low Alc	Hi Alc	Mari- juana	One hard	Two hard
DRGSCORE VALUES	(5)	(12)	(7)	(6)	(9)	(9)
		Percent/(Number)				
Percent having many close friends using alcohol heavily and one illegal drug or two or more illegal drugs	40(2)	0(0)	29(2)	50(3)	56(5)	50(4)

Other Patterns of Association

Consistent with previous research findings, less frequent use of drugs was associated with being married and living with one's spouse (Kandel, 1984). Of the nine members of the sample presently married and living with their spouses, six were using no illegal drugs and using alcohol moderately.

Kandel (1984) also found that high use of drugs was correlated with membership in social networks where high use of drugs was commonplace. This was also true of follow-up respondents. Those consuming more drugs tended to have more close friends also using drugs. Half of those at the high end of the drug score scale reported having many close friends who drank alcohol heavily and used one illegal drug or more, compared to a fourth among those at the low end of the scale. Table 5-12 displays this cross-tabulation which yielded a .26 with Kendall's Tau B, with $p < .02$.

In other respects, those at the high end of the drug scale score showed few differences in their patterns of association from those at low scale positions. All respondents had siblings. No differences were noted in the pattern of sibling interaction among each of the six drug using groups. Those at the high end of the scale were no more likely than those at the low end to have brothers or sisters with experiences of alcohol abuse and/or of any illegal drugs.

However, differences were noted between high and low drug users in the affective relationships respondents had with their siblings. More sibling conflict was noted among those taking more drugs. Table 5-13 displays this relationship which yielded a .21 value with Kendall's Tau B, where $p < .05$. The pattern of increased sibling conflict among those with high drug use seems to be another concomitant of the pattern of living in the parental household and the family conflict that could arise under such circumstances.

Table 5-13.
Drug Abuse and Reporting Conflict/Ambivalent/Indifferent Relations with
One or More Siblings

	None	Low Alc	Hi Alc	Mari- juana	One hard	Two hard
DRGSCORE VALUES	(5)	(12)	(7)	(6)	(9)	(9)
		Percent/(Number)				
Percent with conflict/ambivalent /indifferent relations with one or more sib	60(3)	25(3)	42(3)	17(1)	56(5)	78(7)

Another aspect investigated was former patients' conventional social partic-ipation. A simple seven-point scale was used indicating a person's level of so-cial (and civic) affiliation. Respondents were asked whether they possessed a driver's license, credit card, bank account, library card, voter registration sta-tus, and if they had attended religious services during the past year. No pattern was noted between this civic involvement scale and the drug using scale.

Developing a Predictor Model of the Antecedent Correlates Linked to Post-Treatment Drug Abuse

Based upon the findings in this and the previous chapter, I constructed a pre-dictor model of the antecedent variables in relation to post-treatment drug abuse. One of the factors emerging in the last chapter as a predictor of varia-tions in drug scale scores was age at first use. Those starting to use drugs at earlier ages were more inclined to remain high users at follow-up. The Pearson r between age at first use and drug scale score was .26, p < .08. Age at first use was therefore one of the variables entered in the multiple regression equa-tion.

Time in treatment was also included in the analysis. In the last chapter, time in treatment was found to be the strongest predictor of all the included varia-bles. The range of time in treatment spanned from one month of treatment or less, to as much as one hundred thirty-five months of treatment in day care, therapeutic community, outpatient psychiatric, self-help and other treatments. The Pearson r between time in treatment and drug scale score was .34, p < .02.

Another variable included in the multiple regression equation was whether the respondent had been referred to the Manhasset program by a court order. This information had been obtained from the clinic files. A court referral meant several things. For one, it signified the patient's resistance to getting

Table 5-14.
Court Referral and Drug Abuse Scale Score

	None	Low Alc	Hi Alc	Mari- juana	One hard	Two hard
DRGSCORE VALUES	(5)	(12)	(7)	(6)	(9)	(9)
		Percent/(Number)				
Percent going to treatment by court order	20(1)	42(5)	29(2)	50(3)	67(6)	90(8)

care. It was in response to the court's directive, and not their own inclination, that the individual would participate in treatment. For another, a court order also meant that the respondent had gotten himself in trouble with the law. In many instances those brought into treatment by court orders had committed criminal acts, were apprehended by the police, and courts subsequently had insisted that they receive drug treatment. Another implication of a court order could be that the child was ungovernable. In these cases parents petitioned the juvenile authorities for a court order because they were at wits end with their child. These parents suspected that only with the court order would they be able to stop their child from running away and assure that they remain in treatment. Table 5-14 displays the cross-tabulation between drug scale score and court referral.

I selected the four strongest predictor variables that could be considered as antecedent for multiple regressions in relation to the dependent variable, DRGSCORE. They were as follows: (1) age at first use of drugs; (2) total number of months in treatment; (3) whether patient was referred to treatment by a court order, and (4) whether they lived with parents at follow-up. Together, all the variables yielded an R square of .45. Table 5-15 lists the values of each of the zero-order correlation coefficients, beta weights, F values, significance, and cumulative R squares.

Although each variable contributed something to the total variance explained, living with parents was by far the most decisive of all considered here. When it was omitted from the analysis, the total variance explained dropped from .45 to .26. Multiple regression of these four variables reduced the contributions of age at first use and time in treatment to positions of borderline significance. Thus, court referral and living with parents exerted the greatest influence in explaining variations in post-treatment drug abuse.

There seemed to be a contradiction between the findings presented here and those in the last chapter regarding the significance of time in treatment. Here, multiple regression showed time in treatment to have a modest, if uncertain, influence on the variations in post-treatment drug abuse. While it still contrib-

Table 5-15.
Zero-Order Correlation Coefficients, Beta Weights, F Values, Significance
and Cumulative R Squares

	Zero-order r	Beta weight	F Value	Sig F	Cum. R sq.
1) age at first use	-.26	-.17	1.945	.17	.07
2) months in treatment	-.34	-.17	2.044	.16	.16
3) court referral	.42	.34	8.067	.006	.26
4) now living with parents	.47	.44	14.856	.0004	.45

uted 9% to the total explained variance of drug abuse scores, it failed to achieve statistical significance in the multiple regression. At the zero-order level, however, and among the previously mentioned predictive factors discussed in the last chapter, its impact seemed more substantial. Apparently, it is in concert with these other factors—referral by the courts and living with parents—that its influence builds or diminishes.

Interpretation and Conclusion

In this chapter I examined the correlates of continuing drug abuse among the forty-eight follow-up respondents. Consistent with results of previous research the findings showed increasing drug use to be associated with greater criminal activity, more unemployment, and diminished current educational participation and occupational rank. Those using more drugs reported more psychological problems, especially depression, anxiety, hallucinations, and uncontrollable violence. They were also more likely to be enmeshed in social networks where heavy use of alcohol and illegal drugs was relatively common.

It appears that each of these correlates tends to be mutually supportive. When people are depressed and anxious they may seek drugs to alleviate their distress. Impaired by the effects of drugs, the interest in getting work and the ability to keep a job wanes. Criminal activity increases as those using drugs need money to buy them and provide for their other living expenses. When people are under the influence of drugs they are less inclined to conform to societal norms and inhibit their aggressive impulses. Peer group pressure and peer emulation of other drug users with whom one has social interaction support the interest in drug-taking, the inclination to criminal activity and the aversion to conventional job participation.

This is the vicious cycle of drug abuse that has been well documented by many studies including the present one. One special finding of this research is that the frequent use of two illegal drugs becomes a critical turning point for ushering in a condition where the compound problems associated with drug use are virtually assured. While some of the variables indicated continuous rises with each increasing movement along the drug abuse scale, all of these problem-related correlates became apparent at the point of frequent use of two or more hard drugs.

This follow-up data also documents the possibility of sustaining relatively normal and prosocial adaptations for those engaging in heavy use of drugs but falling short of using two or more hard drugs. Looking at the data closely, it appeared that those taking one hard drug (usually cocaine) less than weekly, in conjunction with heavy marijuana and alcohol use, were able to remain steadily employed compared to others at different use levels. Yet, in examining all the variables linked to the drug abuse syndrome—criminal activities, occupational ranks, psychological problems, association with drug using friends, etc.—the values show this group to be in an intermediate position between those at higher and lower points on each of the variables. While young men in this group outwardly appear to be functioning acceptably in society, they remain extremely vulnerable to joining the ranks of those at the top end of the drug abuse scale. A personal disappointment, a suggestion or urging by a drug-using friend may be all that is needed to arouse a greater use of drugs with all its attendant liabilities.

At the other end of the continuum there is a seemingly surprising incidence of more drug-related difficulties associated with abstinence. When one considers the relatively few numbers of self-directed abstinent respondents one must be especially cautious in generalizing from this particular subgroup. Three of the five respondents were current patients of drug rehabilitation programs and another was under a doctor's care where he received an antidepressant medication. Almost all of these respondents had had recent bouts of heavy drug use which led to their present pursuit of treatment. Current patient status obviously had a lot to do with their abstinence.

It is doubtful that the same trends regarding abstinence would be found in the nonclinic population. I would anticipate that the associations with crime, work, psychological problems, etc. would be much less apparent if nonclinic populations of drug-abstinent white males were being studied. Among a clinic population comparable to the present one, the associated patterns with crime, work, etc. should be very similar to what has been found here. An additional implication of these findings suggests that the awareness of drug-related problems so accentuated among those using two or more hard drugs promotes some functional consequences. Eventually, it seems to inspire some heavy drug users to resume treatment and reduce drug-taking.

One of the more surprising findings uncovered was the correlation between high drug use and living with one's parents. The data suggested that parental enabling and permissiveness may be important in explaining why those living with parents tended to use more drugs. Another possibility may be suggested in the failure to establish satisfactory peer relations which could explain both the pattern of living with parents and engaging in heavy drug use.

Further research, especially with parents, will be needed to more fully understand how living in the parental home encourages high drug consumption. Doubtless, in some homes parental support may have inspired a pattern of low profile drug abuse, sparing the young adult drug user the pursuit of intensive criminality and their eventual detection by the law and treatment agencies. In this mode parents may have established a dependency relationship with their child where intermittent conflict, guilt, hostility, and remorse fuel the urges to take drugs. In other instances parental response may have provided the catalyst for getting the drug-troubled person into care. Future research will need to more deeply probe the structure and relationships of these young adults and their parents to discern the responses that hindered these young men from relinquishing drugs.

Many treatment efforts directed toward reducing adolescent substance abuse, including Manhasset's program, focus on offering treatment to the entire family, conceiving of a patient's abuse problem as a dysfunctionality in family functioning. These results offer confirmation to the appropriateness in applying such theoretical perspectives. Moreover, the findings suggest that family system schemes should be useful in dealing with young adult drug-abusing populations.

In addition, the multiple regression analysis showed continuing drug abuse to have strong links to a person's past. Those getting in trouble with the law as teenagers and resisting clinical intervention—as reflected by court referral to treatment—were inclined to patterns of continuing drug abuse. Starting to use drugs early in life could be an additional, and possibly less important element, in affecting later adult polydrug abuse. Such preceding factors are part of the standard battery of intake questions collected in all governmentally sponsored drug programs. They, therefore, can be readily measured. By identifying those entering patients who are at particular risk for later adult abuse and offering them more diverse and innovative treatments early on, it may be possible to stem the tendencies to recurrent drug abuse. The findings also suggest that more clinical interventions for the preadolescent years will be needed. By the time a youngster is mandated for treatment by the courts, it may already be too late. Such is the conclusion of other recent studies (Kleinman et al., 1987).

The evidence in this chapter may seem to suggest that drug treatments were largely ineffectual in stemming the trend to uncontrolled drug use. While twenty respondents spent a year or more in day care and an additional thirteen more had an average of over three years in various mental health and drug rehabilitation facilities, three-fourths of the follow-up sample were either still heavy drug users at the time of the interview or since they left Manhasset. In this respect many contemporary drug treatments may be regarded as failures for not helping the majority of their potential clientele. Yet, by reducing the numbers of those who use drugs problematically, and by assisting more former abusers to develop prosocial life styles, these programs provide an important service to society. Their abilities to resocialize, however, are evidently short of the miraculous. Given their usually restricted resources, some may be amazed that their rates of successful treatments may be as high as they are.

If the various subgroups in the sample can be identified, this should be helpful for better understanding how treatment benefitted this population. As the sample is subdivided, several different types of user/abuser groups can be distinguished. Among all forty-eight respondents there were approximately 25% of the sample who could be termed greatly improved. These respondents were moderate social drinkers at the time of the interview. During the previous year they worked and/or went to school regularly. Most of these respondents were married and currently living with their spouses. This group reported negligible problems with the law since leaving treatment. They also indicated few psychological difficulties. They were the only respondent population showing evidence of upward mobility in the higher status and better paying positions they held. Most all of these young men expressed great appreciation for their drug treatment experiences. Whether as many would have arrived at their present adaptations without the benefit of therapy remains uncertain. In their perceptions, by and large, the treatment programs were important for promoting their recoveries.

The largest group of respondents, about 45% of sample, were slightly improved. These persons used alcohol and/or marijuana heavily and some were weekend cocaine users. Most all of this group worked steadily, although fewer were going to school and working at white collar jobs, compared with the last mentioned category. These respondents reported more criminal activities and psychological problems than the last mentioned. Yet, few reported heavy post-treatment offense histories or suffered from acute mental stress. No particular living arrangements predominated among this large group of respondents. A few were married and living with their spouses, some lived with girlfriends, others with parents, and some with roommates or by themselves. In contrast to those who were greatly improved, these respondents had shorter treatment experiences. Some had completed treatment programs and felt treatment helped them improve from their earlier daily drug abuse patterns, extreme contentiousness, and depression. Most of these respondents were pleased with their steady employment records and ability to survive without parental assistance. Others had made the rounds to a variety of treatment settings, felt negatively disposed to treatment, and felt it had not helped them much. Some of these individuals felt they outgrew their patterns of drug abuse in spite of the ineffectual professional efforts to help them. Other respondents in this group maintained use patterns that were comparable to their drug consumption levels when they first began Manhasset day care.

Another group of former patients consisted of those whose prognosis seemed uncertain and were "institutionalized" at follow-up. Comprising approximately 10% of the sample, most of these patients abstained from recreational drugs, except for a few moderate social drinkers. Of all the groups in the follow-up population they had the most extensive exposure to drug and mental health treatments. Some were presently under care in residential drug treatment programs or at mental hospitals. When they lived in the community they tended to live with parents or in group homes. Although they reported few psychological problems at the time of the interview (while under care), most indicated a high incidence of problems during the entire aftercare period. There were few who were regularly employed in this group. This subgroup had the highest number of post-Manhasset treatment arrests. These former patients had been through a revolving door of treatments and unsuccessful attempts at living in the community since their initiation into day care. Whether this pattern would persist remained unclear.

The last subgroup among the former day care patient respondents were the unimproved. Numbering about 20% of the follow-up population, these respondents used two or more hard drugs. Most also drank and smoked marijuana heavily. They reported considerable psychological stress and patterns of irregular work. A few were career criminals but more were inclined to a variety of occasional petty crimes. Although they had a range of different living arrangements, most reported living with their parents during the last year. The treatment experiences of this subgroup were varied. Some had been in numerous therapeutic programs, never for long periods of time and usually withdrawing at the earliest opportunity. Others had longer bouts of therapeutic experiences but rarely completed their courses of treatment.

As one considers these diverse subgroups and the preceding cross-tabulation analyses, one can see that treatment reduced the numbers of otherwise unimproved respondents. Yet, the sizable number of persisting drug abusers clearly shows that promoting the retention of those having little motivation to receive care represents one of the most demanding and important challenges that contemporary treatment facilities now face.

6

Conclusions and Overview

The mass media have alarmed Americans about the problem of youth drug abuse. Today's newer drugs, developed and distributed with the aid of our modern technological and transportational resources, have produced difficulties of unprecedented proportions. Many newly synthesized substances, including so-called 'designer' drugs, dispense an unpredictable array of dangerous and toxic consequences when consumed with the more familiar ones. Intravenous drug use—once a risk confined almost exclusively to drug users alone—now presents possibilities of a menacing worldwide epidemic with the spread of the AIDS virus. Cocaine and 'crack' have been added to the assortment of commonly abused drugs; one recent study of a sample of felony arrestees in New York City found an alarming proportion of 90% having traces of cocaine in their urine (Bronstein, 1987). Such evidence suggests that the drug/ crime connection is growing closer with increasing cocaine use. Today more people are beginning to understand that the tragedy of teenage suicide is often preceded by a bout of drug abuse (Wilentz, 1987). These are all new dimensions to youth drug abuse. In the past, such problems either did not exist or were only dimly understood. Today, the trouble-laden implications of youth substance abuse have become much more apparent.

Is youth drug abuse more pervasive today? The perception many share about youth drug use and abuse is that it never was as pervasive as it is now. This supposition is supported by the work of Abelson and Fishburne (1973). In an investigation of a national household probability sample, they found only a fifth of adults twenty-six years of age or older reported ever using an illicit drug, compared to nearly a third of youths aged twelve to seventeen and well over half the young adults aged eighteen to twenty-five. This study documents the spectacular rise in illicit drug use among youth during the 1960s and 70s when many collegians and teens first began experimenting with marijuana and a variety of other psychedelic drugs.

During that time period, marijuana consumption became the dividing point separating the generations of youthful illicit drug users from their elders. By age twenty-five, nearly two-thirds of all interviewed had tried marijuana at least once, but for those over twenty-six only a quarter had ever used the drug (Miller, 1983). Most recently, research evidence is beginning to suggest that

Table 6-1.
Drug Consumption among High School Seniors, 1975 & 1987

	PERCENT EVER USED Class of 1975	Class of 1987
DRUG		
Marijuana	47	50
Inhalants	18 (1979)	19
Hallucinogens	16	10
LSD	11	8
Cocaine	9	15
Heroin	2	1
Other opiates	9	9
Sedatives	18	9
Barbiturates	17	7
Tranquilizers	17	11
Alcohol	90	92
Cigarettes	74	67

(This table was adapted from Table 8, Johnston, O'Malley and Bachman, 1988, pg. 48.)

illicit drug use among teenagers has stabilized or declined somewhat since the mid-70s.

The annual series of systematic, large sample surveys of drug-taking among high school seniors done by the University of Michigan Survey Research Center shows no substantial increases in the numbers using drugs from 1975 to 1987 (Bell and Battjes, 1985; Johnston, O'Malley, and Bachman, 1988). While only a few drugs have gained in popularity over the last twelve years (e.g. cocaine), most others have shown declining use patterns (e.g. LSD, hallucinogens, sedatives, barbiturates, tranquilizers, and cigarettes). Table 6-1 lists the trends in lifetime prevalence for twelve of the most commonly abused drugs.

Evidence from the Michigan Survey Research Center also shows that marijuana use among high school seniors has steadily declined from its peak of 60% in 1979 to 50% in 1987. Some commentators have remarked that today's marijuana smokers are smoking increasingly potent manifestations of the drug compared to what was consumed by earlier generations (Kerr, 1986). Unfortunately, no definitive comparative studies on this question are now possible, but one recent study documents rising concentrations of THC in the marijuana seized by the U.S. Customs Service (Kleiman, 1989).

While illicit drug-taking may be stabilizing or decreasing in some instances, consumption of legal drugs may also be falling. Evidence suggests that the long-term declines in cigarette smoking for all age groups has also been true for teenagers. This is true for males especially. Since the first Surgeon General's report on smoking in 1964, an estimated thirty-seven million Americans have quit the smoking habit (Blakeslee, 1987). Over the duration of their annual series of systematic, large sample surveys of drug-taking among high school seniors, the University of Michigan Survey Research Center reported declining tobacco consumption among high school seniors from 73.6% who (ever) smoked in 1975, to 67.2% in 1987. Daily cigarette consumption also dropped over this same time period from 27% to 19% (Johnston, O'Malley, and Bachman, 1988).

Males, however, experienced the sharpest reductions in cigarette smoking, while female consumption remained more stable. In 1955, 56.9% of all males eighteen years old smoked cigarettes but by 1975 only 39.3% of all males twenty-one years old still smoked. For women, tobacco consumption remained virtually constant. In both 1955 and 1975, some 28% of all women eighteen and older smoked cigarettes (U.S. Dept. HEW, 1970; U.S. Dept. HEW, 1977). As of 1986, the Michigan Survey Research Center group found evidence of greater prevalence of frequent smoking among teenage females than for males (12.5% compared to 10%). In 1975, when the survey first began, males showed the highest cigarette consumption (Johnston, O'Malley, and Bachman, 1988).

Alcohol consumption among youth may have increased during most of the 1970s and may be leveling off or declining slightly during the 80s. Although different studies do not provide entirely equivalent data for long-term comparisons, two studies found youth drinking increased during most of the 1970s. The percent of sixteen to seventeen year olds reporting drinking during the month prior to being surveyed increased from 35% in 1971 to 52% in 1977 (Abelson, Fishburne, and Cisin 1977). Kandel (1980) also reported increasing prevalence of alcohol use among high school students, from 65% to 88% in San Mateo County between 1968 and 1977.

However, longer term, nationwide sample-based surveys conducted by the National Household Survey on Drug Abuse (done at two and three year intervals since 1972) have not confirmed such trends during overlapping time periods (NIDA Capsules, 1986). Owing to differences in use definitions and sampling populations, readers must be wary in comparing findings from disparate investigations. Short-term, or specific locality findings, may not be confirmed in longer-term, nationwide studies. The nationally based Michigan Survey Research Center's annual surveys of high school seniors showed slight rises of occasional heavy drinking among youth from 1975 to 1979 (from 37% to 41% giving such reports), with slight declines to 1975 levels, ever since. In all other respects, they found teenage alcohol use showed remarkable stability from 1975 to 1987.

Since most all of the fifty states have been raising their drinking ages to twenty-one, there is likely to be some reductions in rates of teenage drinking. Wyoming now remains the only exception to the twenty-one year age drinking requirement, whereas in 1979 only fourteen states had such laws (Goode, 1989). One study found alcohol purchases declined by one half among the sixteen to twenty-year-old age group one year after New York State raised its drinking age to twenty-one and use itself declined by 21% (Kolbert, 1987). While the youth drinking prohibition laws are likely to fall far short of their intended aims, they should at least have some impact in stabilizing rates of teen alcohol consumption.

When trying to gauge the changing dimensions of youth drug abuse problems one must be aware of the profound differences between use and abuse. There is a world of difference between the sporadic or experimental consumption of drugs and high frequency use. The former is usually a very normal response and may often represent an important point in the successful transition to adulthood. However, when youngsters take drugs frequently and exhibit compulsive and persistent patterns of drug-taking, it usually represents a sharply contrasting response. In the latter experience individuals are often likely to be in a state of nearly continual conflict with conventional institutions and authority figures. Unfortunately, many of these youngsters tend to drop out of schools prematurely or establish patterns of persistent truancy; consequently, many of these problem-prone youth are not included in school-based drug consumption surveys like the Michigan Survey Research Center's. There are few means to gauge whether the incidence of problematical drug-taking among adolescents has been shifting over the years. Yet, it is by no means trivial to learn that so-called normal drug-taking is showing signs of change. Such fluctuations are likely to have an impact upon problematical drug-taking. Perhaps the most troublesome innovation in so-called normal youthful drug taking today is the introduction of cocaine and crack to the array of commonly used substances. In spite of this, there may be some cause for encouragement in the evidence showing stabilized and declining use of other drugs.

Accounting for the rising patterns of illicit drug use emerging during the late 1960s is an interesting question that bears on our current youth drug abuse predicament. Many have seen the rising illicit drug use linked with the previous period of sociopolitical protest. The civil rights strivings, anti-Vietnam War demonstrations, environment preservation-seeking efforts and other youthful anti-establishment actions also signalled a change in the culturally accepted modes of drug-taking. Many young people began to extol the virtues of marijuana over alcohol. Marijuana became the drug of choice for the youth subculture. For many, it was seen as superior for its absence of hangovers and its apparent fewer adverse health-related effects.

During the 1960s the majority of youthful marijuana users gravitated to its consumption on an occasional and sporadic basis. However, there also emerged growing numbers of heavy drug users who not only used marijuana but also alcohol, as well as a variety of other psychedelic drugs. Such groups of heavier users became known as 'heads;' some were countercultural adherents, deeply disenchanted with American capitalism, consumerism, and the war-oriented economy. For many of the more politically inspired, drug-taking became a political act—dropping out of a society that one found utterly contemptible. Others, of course, as in earlier generations, gravitated to heavier drug use as a way of escaping depression, feelings of inadequacy, and personal problems.

What was important about the rising marijuana and other psychedelic drug consumption of the 1960s was the development of a new culture that was more willing to experiment with a wider variety of psychoactive substances in search of a 'higher consciousness' (Weil, 1972). When books like Carlos Casteneda's *The Teachings of Don Juan: A Yaqui Way of Knowledge* became widely read, and Harvard psychology Professor Timothy Leary became a media celebrity, these were indications that psychedelic drug consumption was becoming approvable conduct, enjoying the support of at least some of society's intellectuals.

Rising youth drug abuse can also be linked to technological developments. Louise Richards (1986) sees drug use as a natural result of human technology. As technology has provided greater opportunities for mood alteration, she claims, society's beliefs have become more accepting of its use. The pharmaceutical industry has been striving to develop new products to cure mental illnesses and to alleviate the anguish of personal distress and pain. As a result there has been a continual accumulation of new drugs, developed and marketed to accommodate the real and imagined medical and psychiatric needs of Americans. Any number of the newer drugs have been synthesized and developed under illegitimate auspices if the legitimate supply sources proved to be too restrictive.

New sedatives, hypnotics, antidepressants, and stimulants have made their appearances and many have become extinct as still newer drugs emerged and became more fashionable. Questions have often been raised about the utility of the drugs and whether doctors were overprescribing them. After a period of critical outcry concerning the overprescription of minor tranquilizers, doctors drastically reduced such prescriptions (Goode, 1989). Two national surveys of legally prescribed psychoactive drugs found only small proportions of persons who overused the drugs or had used them in other than appropriate ways (Mellinger et al., 1978). Yet, questions remain about whether many drug prescriptions now written are actually essential, and whether patients could be helped without the medications.

During the 1960s Marshall McLuhan likened some of the newer psychedelic drugs to a new medium, which could be conceived as an extension of the biochemistry of the body in the metaphorical sense that a computer represented an extension of the brain or nervous system (Lennard et al., 1971). Whether more people today intend to exercise greater control over their moods than in earlier times is an intriguing and highly debatable issue. It is also a question worthy of further research. Nevertheless, the drug technology revolution has placed enormous new powers for mood alteration within people's grasps.

Another basis for widening youth drug abuse has been linked to the weakening of family ties. Some valuable thinking on the subject has been provided by Urie Bronfenbrenner (1967). Bronfenbrenner holds that contemporary suburban living patterns have brought about drastic changes in the family life experience of adolescents. The access that teenagers once had to their parents and to the adult community has been reduced by the advent of the two paycheck family and the fact that fathers often commute long distances to work and mothers have now joined the work force. Extended family ties have also become attenuated as people have moved away from their older urban neighborhoods and the easy informal contact teenagers once shared with other adult intimates. Now, children have been abandoned to suburbia, left to their own resources, to their peer groups, and to the television set. Under these less than adequately structured influences, antisocial conduct, including drug abuse, has been encouraged.

While there has not been any effort to test Bronfenbrenner's overall theory, studies of children's television exposure and diminished parental interaction have shown support for his view in regard to influencing delinquent conduct (Reinhold, 1982; Jessor and Jessor, 1977). However, maternal employment has not been consistently linked to youth antisocial conduct, nor to substance abuse (Nye and Hoffman, 1963). It might be interesting to investigate this theory more fully.

Whatever forces set youthful drug abuse on an increasing course in the 1960s, use levels appear to be stabilizing and even declining in some cases since the middle 70s. However, the associated problems with drug abuse still remain undiminished, if not more troublesome, due to today's widening array of dangerous drugs and their potentially toxic interactive effects.

Societal commitments to reducing drug abuse have historically been very meager. Drug abusers have usually been regarded contemptuously by other members of society. Drug abuse has been seen as a personal failing, the fault of the abuser, and not a matter requiring social attention except to punish abusers for their immoral conduct. Yet, in recent years, in the wake of the current media blitz on drug abuse, governmental appropriations to deal with drug abuse have risen sharply. In 1986, the Congress with President Reagan's support approved a record sum of $1.6 billion in new funds for antidrug programs. As one might expect, the greatest part of this allotment of over a billion dollars was earmarked for law enforcement activities. But, an unprecedented near half billion dollars was appropriated for drug treatment, education, prevention, and research (Brinkley, 1986).

Behavioral scientists have generally shown diminished enthusiasm for law enforcement solutions to problems of drug abuse. Many hold that as long as the demand for drugs remains constant it is simply a matter of time before new underground networks are created to provide for the unsatisfied needs. Most behavioral scientists favor treatment/education/prevention/research efforts because of their potential to reduce desires for drug-taking.

Nevertheless, it seemed that an impressive commitment was being made against drug abuse in the 1986 Anti-Drug Abuse Act. Several months later, however, the act proved illusory when the President cut nearly half a billion dollars off the approved allotments in a budget deficit-cutting mood (Falco, 1987). Thus, the renewed antidrug commitments turned out to be an exercise in political gesturing. Such has been and is the American commitment to reducing drug abuse—unsteadily supported, with a heavily punitive orientation.

Treatment evaluation has been the inspiration for the present study. As has been mentioned before, treatment appears to produce paradoxical results. On the one hand, many studies show that patients remaining in longer-term treatments are inclined to renounce drug abuse and assume more prosocial adaptations. On the other hand, the largest numbers of those entering government-sponsored treatment programs, and especially those whose commitments are made involuntarily, are likely to withdraw and resume drug-taking. Understanding and enlisting the participation of these less receptive clients, who comprise the majority of those now offered treatment, is one of the most troubling problems that drug treatment personnel must confront.

If more successful treatments are to be made, better matchups between clients and the available types of treatments are necessary. Among the different types of programs—whether it be outpatient drug-free, day care, residential treatments, methadone maintenance, or others—it is important to know which kinds of patients, with which kinds of drug problems, and which available family resources, blend together well and enhance the possibilities for program completion and an enduring recovery from abuse.

This strategy was attempted in the present study by identifying the correlates of treatment completion at the Manhasset Community Day Center. The data established that older adolescent patients were more likely to complete the day care program than younger patients. Corroborating earlier studies, there was a trend showing self-referred patients somewhat more inclined to comply with program expectations than those referred by the courts and other outside social agencies, though this fell short of the .05 level of statistical significance. Program completers were less likely to be diagnosed as depressed at intake.

Parental characteristics comprised another group of variables which were related to treatment completion. Parents of higher occupational rank, who had received mental health care for themselves, and of Jewish ethnicity appeared to possess useful strengths for meeting program challenges. Contrary to expectations that parents in intact marriages would find it easier to help their child's treatment progress, the data showed that these parents fared about the same as single parents and parents in reconstituted marriages in having their children succeed in completing care. The pattern of spouse mutuality in dealing with their child's needs, as it existed preceding and during treatment, seemed to be another useful asset for successfully using this form of treatment. While parents with the above characteristics possessed resources that helped them to endure the rigors inherent in this form of care, these attributes also helped project positive images to professional staff about the family and patient's commitments to treatment.

It is important to recognize that although particular identifiable social characteristics were found to be associated with treatment completion, the relations were far from perfect. While patients of certain classes and ethnic affiliations were more inclined to withdraw from treatment programs than others, there are many others who could utilize and benefit from treatment if given the appropriate kinds of inducements and incentives. It is incumbent upon program administrators to recognize that certain groups and individuals may require special additional kinds of care and cultivating efforts if they are to take advantage of available programs. Programs will have to be tailored to meet the diverse sets of needs, abilities, and handicaps that patients and their families present when entering treatment.

As more is learned about the populations attracted and repelled by different treatment programs, administrators will gain considerably. Such information will enhance successes in referring unworkable cases to alternative treatment approaches; it can also encourage a reevaluation and revision of therapeutic requirements maximizing the numbers of persons served.

This research has attempted to establish a starting point for understanding how day care programs help polydrug abusing adolescents. Some of the social characteristics linked with program completion at the Manhasset Day Care program could also be relevant to success in other types of residential and outpatient care. More research will be needed to further delineate the social characteristics linked this and other forms of care for adolescent drug abuse.

Expanding program utilization without diluting basic therapeutic principles comprises an important challenge to program administrators. As program planners confront the diverse and opposing interests among their entering clients, they may often be tempted to shorten the time span for treatment, or to reduce program rules and expectations. Yet, by so doing, they run the risk of creating innocuous courses of treatment in which greater numbers of so-called successful clients will eventually revert to drug use. In the long run a less compromising outlook may provide the richest yield. For those resistant patients, who enter care only as an alternative to incarceration, this research suggests that seeing care work for others may be an important first step in a longer, more torturous course of eventually 'bottoming out,' and then subsequently using therapy to eventually accept help.

Yet, the dilemmas of planning treatment are not always easily rationalized. Sensitive program administrators inevitably face bewilderment and doubt as they reckon with the high client attrition that is inescapable in all governmentally sponsored treatment programs. The large numbers of withdrawing patients often inspires an uneasy mood, giving one cause to wonder whether one may have become too uncompromising in applying treatment philosophies.

Another question explored in this research was the value of day care in combatting teenage multidrug abuse; does it produce any of the benefits claimed for it, such as reduced drug-taking and improved behavioral functioning? Earlier studies have found day care effective in treating alcoholism and narcotic addiction among some adult populations. The evidence accumulated here from the follow-up of former Manhasset patients three to eight years after treatment clearly suggested that day care did help to reduce future drug abuse. Those who spent at least a year or more in care were much less drug-involved than those who withdrew from treatment within six months. Those who were under longer-term care were also much less inclined to be using marijuana and cocaine at follow-up. While long-term patients drank alcohol about as often as dropouts, they tended to drink far more moderately on drinking occasions. The longer-treated group also appeared to be less likely to engage in subsequent criminal activity. They tended to get more schooling and held higher status jobs compared to dropouts, although these differences fell somewhat short of statistical significance. They also reported fewer psychological difficulties and gave more evidence of conventional social participation.

Multiple regression analyses provided additional support to substantiate the relative importance of treatment experience over sociodemographic factors in explaining continuing drug abuse. Whether adolescents started using drugs early in life, their age at treatment and at follow-up, their history of depression, religious backgrounds, parent's social status, drug abuse history, and mental health treatment histories, made less substantial contributions than treatment experience did in accounting for variations in patterns of post-treatment drug abuse.

The evidence supported the utility of day care in treating adolescent multidrug abuse. Day care programs like Manhasset's obviously represent a less costly alternative than residential treatments which also must provide room and board to clients and round the clock professional supervision. Future researchers will find it advantageous to investigate what the actual savings would amount to in running day care versus residential treatment programs.

Of course, there are many adolescent drug abuse clients whose parental resources are so deficient and where interference from drug-using peers is such an ever present threat, that only by removal from their familiar surroundings is it possible to achieve any significant rehabilitative result. Yet, these research results would support efforts toward expanding the availability of day care. By offering day care more widely it should be possible to stretch treatment resources further in serving a larger base of adolescent clientele.

A last part of this investigation focused in depth on the correlates associated with variations in post-treatment drug abuse among the forty-eight former day care patients. Consistent with earlier studies, the results showed increasing drug use associated with more crime, unemployment, and reduced scholastic and occupational attainments. Those using more drugs reported more psychological problems. They were also more likely to have close friends that were heavy and illegal drug users.

Such findings provided support for the value of the DRGSCORE scale as a useful shorthand indicator of drug abuse that could be applied in future drug studies. A trend of rising social difficulties was noted with each different incremental position along the scale, with corresponding rises in the frequency of drug use. The results also suggested that drug users encountered a sharp rise in the numbers of associated problems at the point of consuming two or more hard drugs.

One of the more surprising discoveries was the strong correlation between high drug use and living with one's parents. In the multiple regression analysis, living with parents turned out to be the most decisive factor linked with variations in post-treatment drug abuse. The data suggested that parental enabling and permissiveness may be important in explaining why those living with parents tended to use more drugs.

However, when one considers some of the original precepts of this study, perhaps such findings should not seem all that startling. One of the important underlying themes behind this investigation was an exploration of the importance of the family environment in generating (and relinquishing) patterns of youth drug abuse. The findings have given support to the treatment assumptions applied at Manhasset and elsewhere: family participation and a number of parental and sibling characteristics were linked with treatment completion. In turn, treatment completion was associated with less post-treatment drug use.

Conversely, those parents who could not be sufficiently engaged to conform to treatment center rules would, years later, be inclined to have children who tended to be heavy drug abusers. Most of the former patients that lived with their parents were among those that dropped out of therapy soon after starting and had found the therapeutic expectations irreconcilable with their family life-styles. Their present living arrangements with parents probably intensified the effects of the problematical family elements that may have first brought forth their substance abuse problems.

These results offer confirmation to the appropriateness of conceiving of adolescent drug addiction as symptomatic of a dysfunctional family. Moreover, the findings suggest that family system schemes are not only useful for dealing with adolescent drug-taking, but should also be of value in understanding and treating adult drug-abusing populations.

Most of the adult heavy drug users who lived in their parental homes had long histories of resisting treatment. Of course, in such families not everyone in the household was opposed to getting care. Further research with such families is especially imperative to understand better how those opposed to treatment are eventually able to dominate those amenable to it. Family discord is only one part of the complex gestalt that may lead to a family's premature withdrawal from treatment and their child's persistent drug abuse. Often family members feel uncertainty and doubt about what their problems are; they are often inclined to disavow what the treatment professionals claim as the family's problems.

There are also a great many possibilities prompting both the resistance to taking therapy and the persistence of drug abuse. It seems reasonable to imagine that patterns of parental overprotectiveness, inconsistent rule setting, and indifference would also be important considerations in explaining a young man's persisting drug abuse. In some instances parents may have established dependency relationships with their children where intermittent conflict, guilt, hostility, and remorse fuel the urges of their child to take drugs. Future research will need to more deeply probe the relationships of these young adults and their parents to discern the responses that hindered these young men from taking advantage of treatment and relinquishing drugs.

The evidence obtained here did not show persisting drug abuse related to parental drug abuse patterns. Although other research has yielded some consistent findings showing linkages between parental and child alcoholism, for multidrug abuse the affinities have been less clear (Cloninger et al., 1978; Goodwin, 1979; Goodwin et al., 1977; Halikas and Rimmer, 1974; Kosten, Rounsaville, and Kleber, 1985; Kandel, Kessler, and Margulies, 1978.) Much evidence has shown parental use and abuse of drugs to be subordinate to the influences of peers (Kandel, Kessler, and Margulies, 1978; McCaul et al., 1982; Pederson and Lefcoe, 1985). It may well be that parental substance abuse has a negligible influence in the continuance of multidrug abuse. Again, further research on this issue, with larger samples than the present one, is indicated.

In addition, these findings showed continuing drug abuse to have strong links to a person's past. Those getting in trouble with the law as teenagers and resisting clinical intervention—as reflected by court referral to treatment—were more likely to be continuing drug abusers. Thus, early introduction into drug abuse was linked to later drug problems. These findings are consistent with results obtained by other researchers (Joe and Hudiburg, 1978; Jessor, 1976; Kandel, 1984) .

By identifying those entering patients who are at particular risk for later adult abuse and offering them more diverse and innovative treatments early on, it may be possible to stem the tendencies to recurrent drug abuse. The findings also suggest that more clinical interventions for the preadolescent years will be needed, since by the time a youngster is mandated for treatment by the courts it may already be too late (Kleinman et al., 1987).

In this light, drug use prevention programs can play an important role in insulating youngsters against the persuasive influences of drug-taking peer groups. Botvin and Wills (1985) reviewed a number of school-based evaluational studies that focused on teaching generic personal and social skills to youngsters, helping them to resist invitations and pressure to take drugs. Such recent programs have attempted to avoid the errors of earlier informational oriented, fear arousal approaches which produced little success. Demonstrable results were obtained in a number of experimental programs aimed at reducing cigarette smoking among preadolescents and teenagers (Botvin and Wills, 1985).

Programs that enhance the development of self-esteem and interpersonal competence, which teach adolescents how to resist social pressures to use drugs, which enhance awareness of feelings and the appropriate expression of feelings, which teach stress management and employ positive identification figures can be very helpful in instilling prosocial adaptations among youth (Carroll, 1986). Such programs can become most important for resisting the compelling pressures leading many youth into substance abuse. The further development of such programs holds out some promise for reducing future drug abuse.

Drug Treatment: No Quick Fix

As a concluding note I am reminded of one of the interviews. After covering all the items on the interview schedule one particular respondent told me how difficult he was finding it in his struggle to keep his life in order since his first bout with drugs. He had used a wide range of psychedelic drugs and had been a heroin addict for over two years. He had treatments in a variety of clinical settings—day care, residential treatment, and methadone maintenance. Although he still was bothered by occasional fits of depression, he was extremely pleased with himself for having renounced drugs for more than three years. Now, he was functioning independently of treatment resources, was nearing completion of his undergraduate degree, and supported himself by working nights cleaning out commuter trains. He had aspirations of completing a master's degree in social work and working in the drug rehabilitation field. He looked forward to the time when he would enjoy his work more and have greater economic security.

He remarked how wonderful it would be if there was a drug that could be taken to cure people from their drug problems, swiftly and painlessly. He was most earnest in expressing this solution and said that without it there will never be much progress made in reducing the problem of drug abuse. As I listened I wondered whether it might have been just this kind of unrealistic and magical thinking that helped to instill his earlier dependency on drugs.

Of course, there are no such wonder drugs available; nor can one anticipate such drugs to be available soon, if ever. The path to a drug-free life-style is a tedious and difficult one; it necessarily entails a wholesale change of one's living habits. Temptations to drug-taking usually do not completely disappear. A sense of unremitting struggle, of goals unachieved, occasional depressions and longings for oblivion usually occupy some place in the mind of the ex-abuser. Available treatments usually require continual commitments and renewals of commitment to achieve their intended results. There are no easy and quick treatments, no guarantees of success associated with any kind of care. Treatment is a long and uncertain process; recoveries are tentative and elusive, easily lost to the unchecked urges arising from within the person. Recovery is always sustained by the disciplined effort and resolve made by those who reckon their greater stake (and future benefits) in adhering to conventional practice.

If treatments themselves fall short of the miraculous, so too does the knowledge base that has been accumulated about understanding and improving drug rehabilitation. It is a slow and arduous process, marked with occasional reverses created by the emergence of contradictory findings. Eventually the knowledge base will be expanded, little by little, leading us to a greater comprehension of drug problems and to the recovery from abuse.

It appears that it will be a long time before the high attrition rates found in governmentally-sponsored programs will be reduced. Given that many people enter treatment with little interest in getting care—seeking merely to evade more punitive sanctioning—it seems likely that such unwilling clients will continue to withdraw at their first opportunity. Only after bottoming out, having more anxiety-inducing experiences with drugs and being subject to longer and more confining drug treatments, might they then commit themselves to enduring the discipline inherent in all drug rehabilitation programs.

Appendix A

Codebook for Clinic Files

Variables:

FILE: DEMOGRAF Card 1

1: Identification no. (4) IDNO
2: Age at intake (2) AGEINT
3: Lives with (1) LIVEWITH (Code only one response for each category.
   Always code lowest value when several responses apply).
   codes: 1) with/parents
          2) with/mother only
          3) with/father only
          4) with/other rels.
          5) with/nonkin
          6) with mother and stepfather
          7) with father and stepmother
          8) with both parents and extended kin
          9) with one parent and extended kin
4: Other children at home (1) OTHERKID
codes: 1) only child
       2) has sibs
       3) has sibs and stepsibs
       4) has step sibs only
5: Total number of children in household (2) TOTALKID
6: Patient's dates of birth (4) mo.yr. DOB
7: Age in relation to other children (1) AGESTAT
codes: 1) eldest
       2) middle
       3) youngest
       4) only child
8: Patient's Sex (1) SEX
codes: 1) male
       2) female
9: Sex and Age of other sibs (List up to 6 other sibs; list sex
and age for each with these codes: (1) brother, (2) sister, (3)
younger, (4) older, (0) none (For each sib code sex first, then age).
SIB1 (2)
SIB2 (2)
SIB3 (2)
SIB4 (2)
SIB5 (2)
SIB6 (2)
10: If patient has more sibs than the six above (1) MORSIB
codes: (0) no more sibs
       (1) has more sibs
11: Highest school grade completed (2) GRADCOMP

12: Patient's Race/Ethnic Background (1) RACE
codes: (1) White, not hispanic
       (2) Black, not hispanic
       (3) American Indian
       (4) Alaskan Native
       (5) Asian or Pacific Islander
       (6) Hispanic-Mexican
       (7) Hispanic-Puerto Rican
       (8) Hispanic-Cuban
       (9) Other Hispanic

13: Mothers' Ethnicity as reflected in birthplace (2) MBIRTH
codes: use abbreviations as needed
Two column code for numeric data list:

(01) USA	(13) Greece
(02) Canada	(20) Austria
(03) mexico	(21) Poland
(04) Puerto Rico	(22) Russia
(05) Other No. America	(23) Yugoslavia
(06) South America	(24) Other Europe
(07) England/Scotland	(25) Africa
(08) Ireland	(15) Asia
(09) France	(16) Unknown
(10) Italy	
(11) Germany	
(12) Spain	

14: Fathers' Ethnicity as reflected in birthplace (2) FBIRTH
codes: use abbreviations as needed
Two column code for numeric data list:

(01) USA	(13) Greece
(02) Canada	(20) Austria
(03) mexico	(21) Poland
(04) Puerto Rico	(22) Russia
(05) Other No. America	(23) Yugoslavia
(06) South America	(24) Other Europe
(07) England/Scotland	(25) Africa
(08) Ireland	(15) Asia
(09) France	(16) Unknown
(10) Italy	
(11) Germany	
(12) Spain	

15: Father's occupation (10) FOCCUP

16: Father's occupational rank (1) FOCUPRNK
codes: 1) professional or managerial
       2) white collar, less skilled
       3) skilled manual
       4) semiskilled manual
       5) unskilled manual
       6) unemployed

17: Mother's occupation (10) MOCCUP

17a: mother's activity
     (1) mother working
     (2) mother going to school
     (3) unemployed
     (4) none or no information

18: Mother's occupational rank (1) MOCUPRNK
codes: 1) professional or managerial
       2) white collar, less skilled
       3) skilled manual
       4) semiskilled manual
       5) unskilled manual
       6) unemployed
19: Patient's religion (1) RELIGION
codes: (1) Catholic
       (2) Protestant
       (3) Other Christian (Eastern Orthodox)
       (4) Jewish
       (5) Muslim
       (6) Other Non-christian
       (7) None

20: Previous criminal activities prior to admission (1) PASTCRIM
codes: (1) Serions criminal involvements,e.g. burglary, assault, etc.
       (2) minor criminal offenses, e.g. vandalism, shoplifting, etc.
       (3) none
       (4) juvenile status offenses only (e.g. truancy, running
           away, sexual activities)
21: Prior Arrest(s) (1) PRIORAR
codes: (1) yes (Include PINS Petitions as arrests)
       (2) no
22: When admitted to treatment (4) ADMIT
code: mo.yr.
23: Was patient adopted (1) ADOPT
       (1) Adopted
       (2) Not adopted
       (3) Not reported

24: Age at adoption (2) AGEADOPT
       (01) one year of age or less
       (xx) two digit code for age in yrs.
       (99) not applicable

FILE: DRUGINT   Card 2

23: Nature of referral (1) REFERAL
codes: (1) court-mandated
       (2) mandated by other social agency
       (3) self-referral
       (4) other
       (9) unknown
24: Primary drug use at intake (2) TDRGINT1
codes: (00) none
       (01) heroin
       (02) non-rx methadone
       (03) other opiates and synthetics
       (04) alcohol
       (05) barbiturates
       (06) other sedatives or hypnotics
       (07) amphetamines
       (08) cocaine
       (09) marihuana/hashish
       (10) hallucinogens
       (11) inhalants
       (12) over-the-counter
       (13) tranquilizers
       (14) other
       (15) drug unknown
       (16) PCP
25: Severity of primary drug use (1) SDRGINT1
codes: (1) no use during prior month
       (2) less than once a week
       (3) several times a week
       (4) once daily
       (5) two to three times daily
       (6) more than three times daily
       (7) frequency unknown
26: Secondary drug problem at intake (2) TDRGINT2
codes: (00) none
       (01) heroin
       (02) non-rx methadone
       (03) other opiates and synthetics
       (04) alcohol
       (05) barbiturates
       (06) other sedatives or hypnotics
       (07) amphetamines
       (08) cocaine

```
          (09) marihuana/hashish
          (10) hallucinogens
          (11) inhalants
          (12) over-the-counter
          (13) tranquilizers
          (14) other
          (15) drug unknown
          (16) PCP
27: Severity of secondary drug use (1) SDRGINT2
codes: (1) no use during prior month
          (2) less than once a week
          (3) several times a week
          (4) once daily
          (5) two to three times daily
          (6) more than three times daily
          (7) frequency unknown.

27a: Third drug problem at intake (2) TDRGINT3
codes: (00) none
          (01) heroin
          (02) non-rx methadone
          (03) other opiates and synthetics
          (04) alcohol
          (05) barbiturates
          (06) other sedatives or hypnotics
          (07) amphetamines
          (08) cocaine
          (09) marihuana/hashish
          (10) hallucinogens
          (11) inhalants
          (12) over-the-counter
          (13) tranquilizers
          (14) other
          (15) drug unknown
          (16) PCP
27: Severity of third drug used (1) SDRGINT3
codes: (1) no use during prior month
          (2) less than once a week
          (3) several times a week
          (4) once daily
          (5) two to three times daily
          (6) more than three times daily
          (7) frequency unknown

28: Prior Admission to other programs (1) PRETRET
codes: (1) yes
          (2) no
          (3) unknown
29: School problems prior to admission (1) SCHPROB
codes: (1) no problems indicated
          (2) academic problems only
          (3) academic and discipline problems
          (4) not in school
          (9) not known or reported
30: Patient's mental state at intake (1) MENT
codes: (1) despression indicated
          (2) no symtoms of depression reported
          (9) not known or reported
31: Father's Mental Health Status (1) FMENT
codes: (1) well
          (2) has/had problems and received mental health care
          (3) has/had problems, no care indicated
          (9) Not reported or no information
32: Mother's Mental Health Status (1) MOMENT
codes: (1) well
          (2) has/had problems and received mental health care
```

(3) has/had problems, no care indicated
(9) Not reported or no information
33: Father's drug use/abuse (1) FDRGUS
codes: (1) abuse
(2) uses(d) illegal drugs
(3) high legal use
(4) moderate use of legal drugs
(5) no use of drugs
(9) no information
34: Mother's drug use/abuse (1) MDRGUS
codes: (1) abuse
(2) uses(d) illegal drugs
(3) high legal use
(4) moderate use of legal drugs
(5) no use of drugs
(9) no information
35: Patient's age at first drug use (2) AGEATUSE
36: Parental involvement in managing their child (1) PARMAN
codes: (1) both participate equally
(2) mother more than father
(3) father more than mother
(4) no information reported
(5) single parent household
37: Identification no. (4) IDNO
38: Other child in treatment at program (1) OTHERTRE
codes: (1) yes
(2) no
(3) no information
39: Has sibling(s) with a history of substance abuse problem (1)
SIBDRUG
codes: (1) yes
(2) no
(3) not applicable
(4) no information

FILE: PATPART   Card 3

40: Number of months in program (2) MOSPRO
41: Completion Status (1) COMSTAT
codes: (1) completed or graduated
(2) withdrew or terminated
(3) other
(4) Still in treatment
42: Mother's attendance during treatment (3) TOTALSESM
code: total number of sessions for mother
43: Missed sessions for mother (2) SESMISM
code: total absences for mother
44: Father's attendance during treatment (3) TOTALSESF
code total number of sessions for father
45: Missed sessions for father (2) SESMISF
code: total absences for father
46: Parental drug use became a treatment issue (1) PARDRGPR
codes: (1) yes
(2) no
(3) unknown or not reported
47: Patient cooperation during treatment (1) PATCOOP
codes: (1) much cooperation shown
(2) cooperation generally with some resistence
(3) noncooperation indicated
(4) no information
(5) mixed and uncertain
48: Patient violated program rules during treatment (1) RULVIO
codes: (1) little or no violation of program rules
(2) occasional violation of rules
(3) frequent violation of rules
(9) no information
49: Patient used drugs while in treatment (1) DRGUSTRE
codes: (1) On several occasions or more frequently
(2) rarely

```
          (3) never
          (9) not known
50: Patient committed criminal acts while in treatment (1) CRIMTRE
codes: (1) yes
       (2) no
       (3) patient attempted suicide or showed other serious self
           destructive conduct
       (4) patient committed crime and self destructiveness
       (9) no information
51: Patient left program before finishing treatment (1) LEFTPRO
codes: 1) yes
       2) no
       3) no information
52: Patient referred elsewhere for treatment (1) REFERRED
codes: 1) yes, to residential program
       2) yes, to outpatient program
       3) yes, to other day care or other program
       4) no
       9) no information

53: Primary drug use at discharge (2) DRGDISP
codes: (00) none
       (01) heroin
       (02) non-rx methadone
       (03) other opiates and synthetics
       (04) alcohol
       (05) barbiturates
       (06) other sedatives or hypnotics
       (07) amphetamines
       (08) cocaine
       (09) marihuana/hashish
       (10) hallucinogens
       (11) inhalants
       (12) over-the-counter
       (13) tranquilizers
       (14) other
       (15) drug unknown
       (16) PCP
54: Severity of primary drug use at discharge (1) SDRGDISP
codes: (1) no use during prior month
       (2) less than once a week
       (3) several times a week
       (4) once daily
       (5) two to three times daily
       (6) more than three times daily
       (7) frequency unknown
55: Secondary drug use at discharge (2) DRGDISS
codes: (00) none
       (01) heroin
       (02) non-rx methadone
       (03) other opiates and synthetics
       (04) alcohol
       (05) barbiturates
       (06) other sedatives or hypnotics
       (07) amphetamines
       (08) cocaine
       (09) marihuana/hashish
       (10) hallucinogens
       (11) inhalants
       (12) over-the-counter
       (13) tranquilizers
       (14) other
       (15) drug unknown
       (16) PCP
56: Severity of secondary drug use at discharge (1) SDRGDISS
codes: (1) no use during prior month
       (2) less than once a week
       (3) several times a week
```

      (4) once daily
      (5) two to three times daily
      (6) more than three times daily
      (7) frequency unknown

57: Family relations during treatment (1) FAMRELS
codes: (1) frequent and intense conflict reported
       (2) little and/or infrequent conflict reported
       (3) no information
58: Physical conflict reported (1) PHYSCONF
codes: (1) yes
       (2) no
       (3) no information
59: Parental involvement during treatment (1) PARINVOL
codes: (1) both equally
       (2) father more than mother
       (3) mother more than father
       (4) no information
       (5) neither involved
       (6) single parent household
       (7) mixed and unclear
60: Parental cooperation during treatment (1) PARCOOP
codes: (1) cooperation indicated
       (2) opposition shown
       (3) no information
       (4) father cooperates, mother doesn't
       (5) mother cooperates, father doesn't
       (6) mixed and unclear
61: Mother's behavior during treatment (1) MOBETRE
codes: (1) abnormal behavior indicated e.g. hysterical, anxious,
           withdrawn, angry, guilt ridden, etc.
       (2) normal behavior indicated
       (3) no information
       (4) not applicable
       (5) mixed and unclear
62: Father's behavior during treatment (1) PABETRE
codes: (1) abnormal behavior indicated e.g. hysterical, anxious,
           withdrawn, angry, guilt ridden, etc.
       (2) normal behavior indicated
       (3) no information
       (4) not applicable
       (5) mixed and unclear
63: Identification no. (4) IDNO
64: Patient's family on own initiative pursued other treatment
elsewhere (1) TREELS
codes: 1) yes, 24 hour program
       2) yes, outpatient
       3) yes, other day care or other program
       4) no
       5) no information
65: Staff anticipated that family would get treatment elsewhere
(1) ANTICIP
codes: 1) n/a; patient did not need referral, completed care
       2) family had already entered other program
       3) staff expected family to pursue referral
       4) staff did not expect family to pursue referral
       5) no information

66: Where received previous treatments (7) PASTHELP
codes: use following numbers below in ascending order; use 0 if
did not have that kind of help
1) general or mental hospital
2) outpatient drug rehabilitation
3) residential drug rehabilitation
4) pvt. counselor/therapist, or physician
5) mental health or child guidance clinic
6) school counselor or psychologist
7) self-help group

Appendix B

Youth Treatment Research Project
Department of Sociology
Nassau Community College
Garden City, New York 11530

Identification Number: (4 digits) ____ ____ ____ ____

Current Family Living and Support

1) With whom did you live most of the time during the last year?
   (Code all that apply)
                                            Yes No
Spouse..................................... 1   2
Children................................... 1   2
Parent(s) 1   2
Stepparent................................. 1   2
Other relatives............................ 1   2
Boyfriend or girlfriend.................... 1   2
Other friends.............................. 1   2
Alone...................................... 1   2
Other (specify)_____ 1   2

2) What is your present marital status:
1 Never married
2 married
3 divorced, (If yes, How long? _____ years _____ months)
4 separated, (If yes, How long? _____ years _____ months)
5 widowed, (If yes, How long? _____ years _____ months)

3) How many times have you been married? ____

4) Do you have any children?
   _____ Number

5) How many live with you? _____ number

6) How many people are dependent upon you for support?
   _____ number

7) For each group/person listed below obtain the following
   information:
        A) Has respondent lived with this person during the last
           year?
        B) If respondent has not lived with this person, ask how
           often do they see/phone/or write them?
        C) Ask how they would describe their relationship with this
           person?

With which other family members do you now live? (Use the
following codes below:) (1) Lives with; (2) Does not live with;
(3) Not applicable.

If, does not live with, How often do you get together (or phone or write) with this person? (Use the following codes below:) (1) Once a week or more often;(2) A few times a month; (3) About once a month; (4) A few times a year; (5) About once a year; (6) Never.

How would you describe your relationship to this person? (Use the following codes below:) (1) Positive or good; (2) Mixed; (3) Indifferent; (4) Negative or unpleasant.

PERSON	LIVES WITH	SEES HOW OFTEN	RELATIONSHIP
A Spouse	1 2 3	1 2 3 4 5 6	1 2 3 4
B Child 1st	1 2 3	1 2 3 4 5 6	1 2 3 4
C Child 2nd	1 2 3	1 2 3 4 5 6	1 2 3 4
D Mother	1 2 3	1 2 3 4 5 6	1 2 3 4
4 Father	1 2 3	1 2 3 4 5 6	1 2 3 4
5 Sisters			
a) older	1 2 3	1 2 3 4 5 6	1 2 3 4
b) younger	1 2 3	1 2 3 4 5 6	1 2 3 4
6 Brothers			
a) older	1 2 3	1 2 3 4 5 6	1 2 3 4
b) younger	1 2 3	1 2 3 4 5 6	1 2 3 4
7 Stepparents	1 2 3	1 2 3 4 5 6	1 2 3 4
8 Other relatives			
	1 2 3	1 2 3 4 5 6	1 2 3 4

Social Memberships

8) Age at last birthday   _____

9) What is the highest level of schooling that your father
   completed? (or stepfather if appropriate) (Circle one)
1 Elementary school or less
2 Some high school
3 Completed high school
4 Some college
5 Completed college
6 Post-graduate and/or professional training
7 Don't know or does not apply

10) What is the highest level of schooling that your mother
    completed? (or stepmother if appropriate) (Circle one)
1 Elementary school or less
2 Some high school
3 Completed high school
4 Some college
5 Completed college
6 Post-graduate and/or professional training
7 Don't know or does not apply

11) What is your parents current marital status?
1 Living together
2 One or both deceased (If yes, How old were you when your
   parent died?) ____ years (INTERVIEWER: ask if deceased parent(s)
   was/were divorced or separated. And then fill in below. If both
   parents deceased how old was respondent when second parent died.
   ____ years)
3 parents separated (If yes, How old were you when your
   parent separated?) ____ years
4 parents divorced (If yes, How old were you when your
   parent divorced?) ____ years

Religion

12) What was your religion when you were growing up?
1 Catholic
2 Protestant
3 Other Christian (Eastern Orthodox)
4 Jewish
5 Muslim
6 Other non-Christian
7 None

13) What is your religious preference?
1 Catholic
2 Protestant
3 Other Christian (Eastern Orthodox)
4 Jewish
5 Muslim
6 Other non-Christian
7 None

14) How often do you now go to religious services?
1   Never participate
2   1 - 4 times a year
3   5 - 10 times a year
4   Once or twice a month
5   About once a week
6   More than once a week

Ethnicity

15) Where were you born? (1) U.S. (2) Elsewhere, _____
                                              Specify Country.

16) Where was your father born?
                     (1) U.S. (2) Elsewhere, _____
                                              Specify Country.

17) Where were your fathers' parents born?
        (1) U.S. (2) Elsewhere, _____
                                Specify Countries.

18) Where was your mother born?
                     (1) U.S. (2) Elsewhere, _____
                                              Specify Country.

19) Where were your mothers' parents born?
        (1) U.S. (2) Elsewhere, _____
                                Specify Countries.

Political Affiliations

20) Are you registered to vote in the community in which you now
    live?
1 yes
2 no
3 below voting age/ or not applicable

21) What term best describes your general political preferences?
1 Republican
2 Democratic
3 Independent
4 Other party preference
5 Do not have any particular political preferences

22) Describe the position you usually take on social and political
    issues?
1 Radical
2 Liberal
3 Moderate
4 Conservative
5 None of these terms describe my political sentiments

   In this research we are interested in finding out what has
happened to those who were in treatment or had applied for
admission to the program at Manhasset Community Day Center/
Community House/Project Outreach. We'd like to find out what
you've been doing since you were in treatment.

Education

23) What is the highest degree or diploma you have received?
1 none
2 regular high school
3 General Education Degree (GED)
4 Associates Degree
5 Bachelor Degree
6 Masters Degree
7 Doctoral or advanced professional degree
8 Other (specify:_____)

24) During the last year were you involved in any formal
    educational programs?
1 No
2 part time
3 full time
describe school program

_____
_____

25) In the time period now and when you left the program were you
    involved in any formal schooling experiences?
1 No
2 part time
3 full time
Describe school program

_____
_____

How many years of full time schooling have you completed since you
were involved with this treatment program? _____ years

Employment
26) During the last 12 months how many months have you been
    employed on legitimate jobs (include on the job training as
    employment)?
Full time   _____   months
Part time   _____   months
Been unemployed   _____   months
Attending school
full time   _____   months
part time   _____   months

27) If currently working, what is your position?
    Describe:

----
1 not working
2 going to school
3 working now part time
4 working now full time

28) IF FORMER PATIENT IS MARRIED, then also ask how spouse is
employed. (If not married, then skip to question # 30.

If spouse is currently working, what is his/her position?
Describe:

(Circle all that apply.)
1 not working
2 going to school
3 working now part time
4 working now full time

29) During the last 12 months how many months has your spouse
    been employed on legitimate jobs (include on the job training
    as employment)?
Full time   _____ months
Part time   _____ months
Been unemployed   _____ months
Attending school
full time   _____ months
part time   _____ months

30) Altogether, how many weeks did you work or go to school in the
last 12 months? _____ weeks

31) If working, what is your current annual gross salary? (Show
card).
1 under $10,000
2 between $10,001 and $20,000
3 between $20,001 and $30,000
4 between $30,001 and $40,000
5 between $40,000 and $50,000
6 over $50,000

32) What is the approximate total annual gross income of the
household where you are now living?
Household Income (Show card)
1 under $10,000
2 between $10,001 and $20,000
3 between $20,001 and $30,000
4 between $30,001 and $40,000
5 between $40,000 and $50,000
6 over $50,000

Social Participation

33) Does respondent possess:
A) Driver's license   (1) Yes (2) No
B) Bank account   (1) Yes (2) No
C) Credit card   (1) Yes (2) No
D) Library card   (1) Yes (2) No

34) During the last month about how many hours would you say you spent with close friends socializing?

1) 10 or less hours
2) between 11 and 25 hours
3) over 25 hours
4) unable to answer

Physical and Mental Health

35) How many times in your life have you ever been hospitalized for medical problems? (INCLUDE ALL HOSPITALIZATIONS)

---- ----

36) How many times in your life have you ever been hospitalized for OD's or DT's ?   ---- ----

37) How many times in your life have you ever been hospitalized for detoxification?   ---- ----

38) How many times since you were involved with the treatment facility were you hospitalized for OD's, DT's or detoxification?   ---- ----

39) What was the total time you spent in a hospital for a physical problem since you left/completed treatment at the MCDC/CH/PO facility?   ---- ---- months   ---- ---- days

Interviewer: Use scrap paper to go over with respondent each of all hospitalizations that patient had since treatment and put totals in for item 39.

40) Do you have any chronic medical problems which continue to interfere with your life? 1 Yes   2 No

41) Are you taking any prescribed medication on a regular basis for a physical problem? 1 Yes   2 No

42) During the last month, on how about many days have you experienced medical problems?   ---- ----

43) In the last 3 months how often have you been to a doctor?
1 Never
2 Once
3 Twice
4 3-5 times
5 more often

44) In your life how many times (different episodes of treatment) have you been treated for any psychological or emotional problems?

---- ---- Total number of times?
---- ---- In a hospital?
---- ---- As an outpatient or private patient?

How many times were you treated for any psychological or emotional problems since you withdrew or completed treatment at MCDC/CH/PO?

---- ---- times
---- ---- In a hospital?
---- ---- As an outpatient or private patient?

45) Have you had a **significant** period, (that was not a direct
result of drug/alcohol use) in which you:
(Use these codes: (0) No   (1) Yes)

	Past 30 Days	In your Life
A Experienced serious depression	____	____
B Experienced serious anxiety or tension	____	____
C Experienced hallucinations	____	____
D Experienced trouble understanding, concentrating or remembering	____	____
E Experienced trouble controlling violent behavior	____	____
F Experienced serious thoughts of suicide	____	____
G Attempted suicide	____	____

46) How many days in the past 30 have you experienced any serious
    psychological or emotional problems?   ____

47) Most of the time since treatment at MCDC/CH/PO have you had
    regular access to a car?
(1) no
(2) occasionally or periodically
(3) regularly

48) Were you ever involved in an accident where you or someone
    else was seriously injured? (1) Yes   (2) No

If yes: What kind? _____   How many times? _____ times

When did this occur? (Use the following codes below:)
(1) Before treatment; (2) During treatment; (3) After treatment

Any other accidents? How many accidents altogether? (Enter
responses below.)

For each accident mentioned, fill in information here:
Type of Accident   When occurred
1)_____   1   2   3

2)_____   1   2   3

3)_____   1   2   3

4)_____   1   2   3

5)_____   1   2   3

49) How many places have you lived in during the last year? ____

PRESENT DRUG USE

50) During the last two months on the average how often have you
    drunk beer, wine or liquor?
1) Not at all
2) less than once a week
3) on several days during a week
4) daily

51) On days that you drink about how many drinks do you usually
have?
Show card saying that one drink = 12 oz. bottle of beer = 4 oz.
wine = or 1 and 1/3 oz. of liquor
_____ drinks

52) During the last year have you had any of the following:
Blackouts 1) yes 2) no
Hangovers 1) yes 2) no
Loss of apetite or stomach distress 1) yes 2) no
Being drunk 24 hours or more at a time 1) yes 2) no

53) During the last year has excessive use of alcoholic beverages
    ever caused trouble in the following areas:
Work or school studies 1) Yes 2) No
Relations with family or friends 1) Yes 2) No
Health 1) Yes 2) No
The law 1) Yes 2) No
Finances 1) Yes 2) No

54) What drugs did you use during the last two months?
(Ask about each category of drugs separately.)
(Use frequency code below for each item and list in LEFT BOX.)
(1) Daily; (2) Several times a week; (3) less than weekly;
(4) not at all
(INTERVIEWER: If any drugs were used, then ask:) Did this drug
cause you any problems in any of the following areas:
A) work or school studies; B) health; C) criminal activities to
get money; D) forgoing food for drugs; E) aggressive or wild
behavior
(For each drug consumed, use the RIGHT column to list the letters
of all areas where former patient had problems. If patient had no
problems write "None" in each box.)

	Frequency	Problems
Heroin	____	____
Methadone (illegal)	____	____
Other Opiates	____	____
Barbituates, sedatives, tranquillizers	____	____
Cocaine	____	____
Amphetamines and similar agents	____	____
Hallucinogens (LSD, mescaline, peyote, etc.)	____	____
Marijuana	____	____
Inhalants	____	____
Other: _____	____	____
specify		

Arrest History

55) Were you ever arrested by the police?
1 Yes
2 No

If Yes, what were the charges and when was this in relation to
treatment at the MCDC/CH/PO program?
1 Before treatment
2 During treatment
3 After treatment

List responses below:

Arrests or criminal charges   When in relation to drug treatment

First time: _____   1 Before   2 During   3 After

Second time: _____   1 Before   2 During   3 After

Third time: _____   1 Before   2 During   3 After

Fourth time: _____   1 Before   2 During   3 After

Fifth time: _____   1 Before   2 During   3 After

Sixth time: _____   1 Before   2 During   3 After

Review charges mentioned above and record next to categories
below. So you were charged ____ times with _____ (crimes), does
that seem correct? Have you ever been arrested or charged with any
of the following? Continue until all charges are coded below.

Number of times
charged

Crimes against persons--e.g.,assault,
rape, battery, homicide, manslaughter................_____

Crimes of profit--e.g., stealing, armed
robbery, robbery, burglary, forgery, theft,
keeping money under false pretenses.................._____

Drug violations--e.g., dealing, possession.........._____

Prostitution, pimping or soliciting................._____

Other (including minor offenses, DWI, reckless
driving, vagrancy, disorderly conduct, public
intoxication, etc.) ...._____

56) How long did you spend in jail for any of these offenses?
    (Put down totals here:)   _____ years ____ months

57) Have you done any of these below listed things during the last
two months for which you were NOT charged by the police?

a) Have you done any of the things in category (I) in the last two
months. Just say yes or no.
b) Have you done any of the things in category (II) in the last
two months. Just say yes or no. INTERVIEWER: Go from III through
VI with the same set of questions.

                                                     Yes   No
I   - Shoplifting, pickpocketing or burglary....... 1   2

II   - Purse snatching, armed robbery, forgery,
          auto theft, blackmail, or extortion.......... 1   2

III   - Arson, vandalism or other damaging
          of property.....................................1   2

IV   - Assault, battery, mugging, rape...............1   2

V   - Soliciting, pimping, prostitution.............1   2

VI – Dealing in drugs, forging prescriptions,
       stealing drugs...............................1   2

AFTER TREATMENT THERAPY

58) After leaving or completing this treatment program, did you
receive treatment in any of the following places:

A) A METHADONE MAINTENANCE PROGRAM?   (1) Yes   (2) No

How many times did you enter such a program?   _____

Total number of months received treatment there _____

B) A THERAPEUTIC COMMUNITY PROGRAM?   (1) Yes   (2) No

How many times did you enter such a program?   _____

Total number of months received treatment there _____

C) A DETOXIFICATION PROGRAM?   (1) Yes   (2) No

How many times did you enter such a program?   _____

Total number of months received treatment there _____

D) AN OUTPATIENT DRUG FREE PROGRAM?   (1) Yes   (2) No

How many times did you enter such a program?   _____

Total number of months received treatment there _____

E) ANOTHER DAY CARE PROGRAM? (1) Yes   (2) No

How many times did you enter such a program?   _____

Total number of months received treatment there _____

59) After leaving or completing this treatment program, did you
receive treatment for drug use or other problems from any of the
below mentioned persons:

A) Psychiatrist, psychologist, or social worker: (1) yes (2) no
   If treated: How long did treatment last? _____ months

B) If yes to above was it, group or individual counseling?
(1) individual; (2) group; (3) both individual and group therapy;
(4) not applicable.

C) priest, rabbi, or other clergyman: (1) yes (2) no
   If treated: How long did treatment last? _____ total no. months

D) Family physician: (1) yes (2) no
   If treated: How long did treatment last? _____ total no. months

E) Community or self help counseling group: (1) yes (2) no
   If treated: How long did treatment last? _____ total no. months

60) How long has it been since your last treatment/counseling/
group therapy experience? _____ months

FEELINGS ABOUT VALUE OF THERAPEUTIC EXPERIENCES

61) People have different reasons for going into drug treatment.
How important were each of the following reasons when you went
into treatment at the program. READ THROUGH ALL THE REASONS. For
you, was it very important, somewhat important, not too important,
or not at all important?

	Very important	Somewhat important	Not important at all
a) you had pressure from a parole or probation officer.....................3	2	1
b) you had legal problems and treatment was required or advised by police/courts/ lawyers/etc................3	2	1
c) your family wanted you to.....................3	2	1
d) your friends wanted you to................... 3	2	1
e) drugs were hard to get or unavailable............3	2	1
f) the quality of drugs was poor.......................3	2	1
g) you had medical or physical problems..........3	2	1
h) you decided for yourself that you wanted treatment..3	2	1

62) At that time was the program very easy for you to travel to,
fairly easy, or hard? ____
1) Very easy
2) Fairly easy
3) Hard

63) Did you feel that most of the treatment staff you knew there
perform their jobs very well, pretty well, or not well as far as
you could tell? ____
1) Very well
2) Pretty well
3) Not well
4) don't know

64) Did you gain a lot of understanding of your drug problems,
some understanding, or not much understanding, as a result of
treatment at that time?
1) A lot of understanding
2) Some
3) Not very much

65) Did the staff there try to help you with other kinds of
problems in your life, or did they work only on drug problems?
1) Other kinds of problems too
2) Only drug problems
3) Don't know

66) Did you feel that any of the staff there cared about you as an
individual and how your life turned out?
1) Yes
2) No
3) Don't know

67) Did you feel that the individual treatment you got at the
program was:
1) too much
2) just about right
3) not enough
4) don't know

68) Were you satisfied with the drug treatment you received there,
somewhat satisfied, or not at all satisfied?
1) Very satisfied
2) Somewhat satisfied
3) Not at all satisfied
4) Don't know

69) Was there anything you particularly liked about the drug
treatment program?
1) Yes
2) No
If Yes: What did you particularly like?
RECORD VERBATIM

_____

_____

70) Were there anythings you particularly disliked about the
program?
1) Yes
2) No

If Yes: What did you particularly dislike?
RECORD VERBATIM

_____

_____

71) If withdrew, explain why you left the program
_____

_____

_____

_____

_____

72) Here are some of the complaints clients have had about various drug programs. These don't necessarily apply to the program you were in at Manhasset/Community House/Project Outreach. However, I would like to know if any of these apply to your experience at the program.

	not a problem	small or some problem	big problem
Too little contact with doctors or psychiatrists....1	2	3
Too little privacy--you couldn't get away from the other clients...............1	2	3
Too boring, not enough to do............1	2	3
Too many unnecessary rules..1	2	3
Not treated with respect by staff....................1	2	3
Not enough staff............1	2	3
Illicit drugs available.....1	2	3
Clients were kept in treatment too long..........1	2	3
Clients were made to leave treatment too early.........1	2	3
Too little opportunity for group therapy...............1	2	3
too little opportunity for individual therapy or counseling..................1	2	3

73) Being in a drug program can help clients in a lot of different ways. Did being in the program at Manhasset/Community House/Project Outreach during the time you were in treatment help you in any of the following ways? IF RESPONDENT ANSWERS NO, ASK: "Did you need that kind of help when you were there?"

	Yes	No, but Not needed	No, and Needed
1) Did the program reduce your use of the drug you were being treated for?...........1	2	3
2) Did the program get you off the drug you were being treated for?...........1	2	3
3) Did the program help you get off drugs other than your main drug of abuse?.....1	2	3
4) Did the program help you stay out of jail?............1	2	3

5) Did the progam help your
state of mind, help you
feel better, less depressed?.1   2   3

6) Did being in the program
get you help with a physical
health problem?..............1   2   3

7) Did the program help you
to reduce your drinking?.....1   2   3

8) Did the program help you
to reduce your smoking?......1   2   3

9) Did the program give you an
opportunity to make new
friends you still have?......1   2   3

10) Did the program give you
an opportunity to get more
education or training than
you would have otherwise?....1   2   3

11) Did the program help you
to get along with other
people better?...............1   2   3

74) Considering your experiences in this drug program, how would
you rate the importance of each the following people or groups in
helping you give up drugs.

	Very important	Somewhat important	Not important at all
A) Other patients in the program	3	2	1
B) "High Hats," high status patients in treatment	3	2	1
C) The counselor(s) I worked with	3	2	1
D) staff members at the center who had been ex-addicts	3	2	1
D) All the people employed at the center that worked with me.	3	2	1
E) My parents	3	2	1
F) My brothers and sisters	3	2	1
G) Family therapy or treatment sessions	3	2	1
H) Probation/parole officer	3	2	1

75) Can you think of any parts of the program that stand out in your mind as being especially important in helping you stay away from drugs?

_____

_____

76) Can you think of any parts of the program that stand out which created a setback to you in your efforts to give up drugs?

_____

_____

77) How would you rate the cooperation of your family in your treatment at the program?
(1) They couldn't have helped more in my treatment.
(2) They helped somewhat but they could have done more.
(3) They neither helped nor hindered the treatment.
(4) They hindered the treatment.

78) How would you rate the requests and expectations of professional staff at the program for your family's support?
1) they expected too much of my family
2) they expected the right amount of help and involvment
3) they could and should have gotten more cooperation from my family.

ROLE OF FAMILY IN THE TREATMENT EXPERIENCE

79) At the time you received treatment from the program which family members were you living with? (See list below.)

How would you rate each in helping you succeed in the program?
1) Helped a lot or a great deal
2) helped somewhat
3) neither helped nor hindered me
4) interfered somewhat with my treatment
5) interfered a great deal with my treatment

How would you describe each person's use of drugs and/or alcohol while you were in treatment:
1) Used drugs/or alcohol heavily or frequently
2) Used drugs/or alcohol moderately
3) Abstained from using drugs/or alcohol altogether

INTERVIEWER: Enter these responses below:

	Role in Helping	Drug Behavior
Mother		
(1) yes (2) no (3) not applicable	1 2 3 4 5	1 2 3
Father		
(1) yes (2) no (3) not applicable	1 2 3 4 5	1 2 3
Stepmother		
(1) yes (2) no (3) not applicable	1 2 3 4 5	1 2 3
Stepfather		
(1) yes (2) no (3) not applicable	1 2 3 4 5	1 2 3
Older brother(s)		
(1) yes (2) no (3) not applicable	1 2 3 4 5	1 2 3
Younger brother(s)		
(1) yes (2) no (3) not applicable	1 2 3 4 5	1 2 3

Older sister(s)
(1) yes (2) no (3) not applicable 1 2 3 4 5   1 2 3
Younger sister(s)
(1) yes (2) no (3) not applicable 1 2 3 4 5   1 2 3
Other relative(s)
(1) yes (2) no (3) not applicable 1 2 3 4 5   1 2 3

80) Overall how would you rate the support you received from your
entire family in your drug treatment involvement at the center.

Select a number from 0 to 4, with 4 as the most support
imaginable, and 0 as the most possible interference. _____
0 Great interference
1 Some interference
2 neutral
3 Some help and support
4 Great help and support

Family Drug Use

81) Up until you were 16 years old, did you always live with your
mother and father?
1 yes 2 no

82) How would you describe your father's use of alcohol during the
time you were growing up?
1 Never drank
2 Light drinker
3 Moderate drinker
4 Heavy drinker
5 Very heavy drinker

83) How would you describe your father's use of alcohol during the
last three years?
1 Never drank
2 Light drinker
3 Moderate drinker
4 Heavy drinker
5 Very heavy drinker
6 Can't answer or don't know

84) How would you describe your mother's use of alcohol during the
time you were growing up?
1 Never drank
2 Light drinker
3 Moderate drinker
4 Heavy drinker
5 Very heavy drinker

85) How would you describe your mother's use of alcohol during the
last three years?
1 Never drank
2 Light drinker
3 Moderate drinker
4 Heavy drinker
5 Very heavy drinker
6 Can't answer or don't know

86) Has your father used any of the following drugs for
non-medical reasons?

INTERVIEWER: Use the following categories:
Use: (1) yes; (2) no; (3) don't know
Frequency: (1) Often; (2) occasionally; (3) once or twice; (4) never
If known that parent used drug in last three years put a check in box at right.

	Used drug			Frequency				Used last 3 years
A) marijuana or hashish:	1	2	3	1	2	3	4	____
B) LSD or other psychedelics:	1	2	3	1	2	3	4	____
C) methedrine ("speed"):	1	2	3	1	2	3	4	____
D) "ups"--amphetamines:	1	2	3	1	2	3	4	____
E) "downs"--barbituates:	1	2	3	1	2	3	4	____
F) tranquilizers:	1	2	3	1	2	3	4	____
G) cocaine:	1	2	3	1	2	3	4	____
F) heroin:	1	2	3	1	2	3	4	____
G) inhalants:	1	2	3	1	2	3	4	____

87) Has your mother used any of the following drugs for non-medical reasons?

INTERVIEWER: Use the following categories:
Use: (1) yes; (2) no; (3) don't know
Frequency: (1) Often; (2) occasionally; (3) once or twice; (4) never
If known that parent used drug in last three years put a check in box at right.

	Used drug			Frequency				Used last 3 years
A) marijuana or hashish:	1	2	3	1	2	3	4	____
B) LSD or other psychedelics:	1	2	3	1	2	3	4	____
C) methedrine ("speed"):	1	2	3	1	2	3	4	____
D) "ups"--amphetamines:	1	2	3	1	2	3	4	____
E) "downs"--barbituates:	1	2	3	1	2	3	4	____
F) tranquilizers:	1	2	3	1	2	3	4	____
G) cocaine:	1	2	3	1	2	3	4	____
F) heroin:	1	2	3	1	2	3	4	____
G) inhalants:	1	2	3	1	2	3	4	____

88) Did you ever get any illegal drugs from your parents?
(1) No
(2) yes, sometimes
(3) yes, often

89) If yes to above: Did parents know you had some of their drugs?
(1) Parents did not know
(2) Parents knew, but had not offered drugs to patient
(3) Parents knew, and had offered drugs to patient

90) Would you say that many of your parents' close friends "get high" (use illegal drugs or take legal drugs for non medical uses)?
(1) No
(2) a few may, but not most of their close friends
(3) Yes

91) How many of your brothers and sisters have had problems from drinking too much alcohol or taking other drugs? _____

92) Were any of your brothers heavy drinkers? (1) Yes; (2) No; (3) don't know.

93) Have any of your brothers had drinking problems during the
last three years? (1) Yes; (2) No; (3) don't know.

94) Were any of your sisters heavy drinkers? (1) Yes; (2) No; (3)
don't know

95) Have any of your sisters had drinking problems during the last
three years? (1) Yes; (2) No; (3) don't know.

96) Have any of your brothers ever used any of the following drugs
for non-medical reasons?

INTERVIEWER: Use the following categories:
Use: (1) yes; (2) no; (3) don't know
Frequency: (1) Often; (2) occasionally; (3) once or twice; (4)
never
If known that a brother used this drug in last three years put a
check in box at right.

	Used drug	Frequency	Used last 3 years
A) marijuana or hashish:	1 2 3	1 2 3 4	____
B) LSD or other psychedelics:	1 2 3	1 2 3 4	____
C) methedrine ("speed"):	1 2 3	1 2 3 4	____
D) "ups"--amphetamines:	1 2 3	1 2 3 4	____
E) "downs"--barbituates:	1 2 3	1 2 3 4	____
F) tranquilizers:	1 2 3	1 2 3 4	____
G) cocaine:	1 2 3	1 2 3 4	____
F) heroin:	1 2 3	1 2 3 4	____
G) inhalants:	1 2 3	1 2 3 4	____

97) Have any of your sisters ever used any of the following drugs
for non-medical reasons?

INTERVIEWER: Use the following categories:
Use: (1) yes; (2) no; (3) don't know
Frequency: (1) Often; (2) occasionally; (3) once or twice; (4)
never
If known that a sister used this drug in last three years put a
check in box at right.

	Used drug	Frequency	Used last 3 years
A) marijuana or hashish:	1 2 3	1 2 3 4	____
B) LSD or other psychedelics:	1 2 3	1 2 3 4	____
C) methedrine ("speed"):	1 2 3	1 2 3 4	____
D) "ups"--amphetamines:	1 2 3	1 2 3 4	____
E) "downs"--barbituates:	1 2 3	1 2 3 4	____
F) tranquilizers:	1 2 3	1 2 3 4	____
G) cocaine:	1 2 3	1 2 3 4	____
F) heroin:	1 2 3	1 2 3 4	____
G) inhalants:	1 2 3	1 2 3 4	____

98) Below are listed a number of statements about relationships
children sometimes have with their parents. For each statement
indicate whether this is true about how you got along with your
parents when you were a teenager.

	Strongly agree	Somewhat agree	Somewhat disagree	Strongly disagree	Don't know
A) My parents were very strict with me.	1	2	3	4	5

B) They set
definite rules
for controlling
and deciding
things you could do.
          1   2   3   4   5
C) Whether I did
good or bad, my
parents never seemed
to be very interested.
          1   2   3   4   5

D) They were consistent
from one time to another
in the rules and decisions
made for you. 1   2   3   4   5

E) They wanted you to
learn to make your
own decisions as you
grew older.   1   2   3   4   5

F) My parents were
often preoccupied with
their own activities
and involvements and
rarely showed much
concern for me.
          1   2   3   4   5

G) There were serious
arguments or fights
between you and
your parents. 1   2   3   4   5

H) They seemed to trust
and understand you.
          1   2   3   4   5

I) They knew who
you were with and
what you were doing
when you weren't
at home.   1   2   3   4   5

J) They had serious
arguments and fights
with one another, or
others in your family.
          1   2   3   4   5
K) Your family spent
a lot of time doing
things or going
places together.
          1   2   3   4   5
L) You had responsibilites
or things you had to
do as part of your
family.   1   2   3   4   5

M) Whenever I had a problem
--school or personal--I've
always felt that my
parents would be interested,
and helpful to me.
                    1   2   3   4   5

N) Because of their excessive
interest in me, I sometimes felt
my parents didn't really want
to see my grow up and
be on my own. 1   2   3   4   5

O) My parents often interfered
in my life and told me
what to do.   1   2   3   4   5

99) How were you usually punished as a child?

1) Physically punished
2) reprimanded verbally, or deprived of something
3) told how you should have acted
4) warned not to do it again, but seldom punished
5) sent to bed

100) For each of these drugs listed, please tell me how many of
your present close friends use them fairly regularly.

	None	A few	Many
A) Marijuana	1	2	3
B) Heroin	1	2	3
C) Barbituates	1	2	3
D) Cocaine	1	2	3
E) Amphetamines	1	2	3
F) Hallucinogens	1	2	3
G) Heavy use of alcohol	1	2	3

    Thank you very much for all your generous cooperation in
answering all these questions and in giving us so much of your
valuable time. If you would like a copy of our findings please let
me know now and I will make sure the research director adds your
name to the list of those who will be receiving final study
reports.

Interviewer Impressions Information

TO BE FILLED OUT AFTER COMPLETING INTERVIEW

1) Do you think your respondent's answers to the questions were in any way evasive? If yes, please explain.

----

2) Were there any particular topics discussed where respondent answered evasively? List below those places.
----

3) Did you detect any inconsistencies in the pattern of answers. Please explain below.

----

4) Were there any other reasons to suspect that questions were not answered truthfully? Please explain and indicate which information is potentially untrue or unreliable.

----

5) Did the person's physical appearance (e.g. eyes, nose, face) and motor behavior suggest drug use or misrepresentation of their present activities. If yes, please explain.
----

6) Did person's grooming and clothing look especially disorderly or in disarray.
If yes, please explain.

----

7) Was the home setting especially dirty, disorganized or chaotic. If yes, please explain briefly.

----

8) Did the person's mental state appear rational and coherent? If not, please explain briefly.

----

9) Was patient overly suspicious? If yes, please explain.

Appendix C

LONG ISLAND JEWISH—HILLSIDE MEDICAL CENTER • NEW HYDE PARK, NEW YORK 11042   (212) 470-2406,2407

M.D., M.P.H., F.A.C.P.M.
CHAIRMAN, DEPARTMENT OF COMMUNITY MEDICINE

PROFESSOR OF COMMUNITY MEDICINE
SCHOOL OF MEDICINE
HEALTH SCIENCES CENTER
STATE UNIVERSITY OF NEW YORK AT STONY BROOK

Name
Address
Town, State, Zip

Dear Mr. Name :

    As you know, throughout the years, Long Island
Jewish-Hillside Medical Center, has provided many services to
residents of Nassau County. Although at times it is not difficult
to realize the value of our services, at other times we don't know
how much help our programs have offered to the people who received
them.

    We are presently trying to locate and interview people who
had contact with some of the hospital's programs in the past. It
is our understanding that you availed yourself of services in one
of these programs now under study.

    We would like the opportunity to have a member of the faculty
of Nassau Community College, Professor William Feigelman, or a
member of his research staff, arrange an interview with you at
your convenience in the near future. We are hoping that you will
cooperate in this effort when you are contacted. The information
you provide is extremely vital in our efforts to better understand
and improve the quality of services we offer to citizens of Nassau
County.

    Please let me assure you that the information you contribute
will be strictly confidential and will only be used for
statistical purposes.

    This research is being conducted in compliance with federal
informed consent regulations. Your participation is completely
voluntary. You may refuse to cooperate with all or any part of the
interview that you may wish to. Your participation or
nonparticipation in the study will not any way effect your
opportunities to receive future treatment from the hospital.

                        Sincerely,

                            M.D., M.P.H., Chairman,
               Department of Community Medicine

CLINICAL CAMPUS OF THE HEALTH SCIENCES CENTER, STATE UNIVERSITY OF NEW YORK AT STONY BROOK

Appendix D

Summary of Results: Clinic Files Analysis

	Completed Program		Time in Treatment (yr. or more vs. less)	
	X^2	p	X^2	p
1) Age	5.98	.05	1.92	.38
2) Age at First Use	8.39	.038	5.75	.12
3) Father's Occup. rank	6.27	.036	1.80	.40
4) Ethno-religious	13.44	.001	3.91	.40
5) Father's Drug Abuse	2.18	.139	.308	.57
6) Mother's Drug Abuse	3.15	.53	7.84	.44
7) Father's mental health/treatment status	3.12	.21	5.40	.06
8) Mother's mental health/treatment status	8.59	.01	12.54	.01
9) sex	.146	.70	1.578	.45
10) Prior treatment experience	.288	.59	.536	.76
11) Prior criminality	2.05	.15	1.81	.17
12) Depression	8.05	.004	3.63	.05
13) Self-referral	3.19	.073	1.48	.22
14) Family structure/ Divorce	4.81	.68	10.49	.72
15) Only child living at home	.889	.34	8.97	.002
16) Sibling rank	.12	.98	.527	.76
17) Adopted Status	.01	.92	2.28	.32
18) Other sibling in treatment at center	2.015	.15	6.81	.033
19) Sibling w/substance abuse history	.547	.45	3.35	.19
20) Older brother at home	4.167	.05	11.008	.20
21) Frequency of use of chiefly abused drug	2.33	.126	.517	.47
22) Abuse of hard drugs	.340	.56	.038	.98
23) Number of drugs abused	2.18	.53	1.595	.95
24) Father's participation	48.693	.000	156.61	.000
25) Mother's participation	45.551	.000	223.11	.000
26) Shared parental involvement	20.53	.000	33.21	.000
27) Parental mutuality (at intake)	9.00	.002	3.97	.046
28) Parental cooperation during treatment	28.48	.000	32.32	.000
29) Mother's behavior during treatment	5.091	.02	5.64	.05
30) Father's behavior during treatment	4.99	.02	7.36	.02
31) Parental abstinence during care	.11	.73	.007	.92
32) Family conflict	25.38	.000	17.65	.000
33) Physical family conflict	4.83	.02	4.80	.09
34) Crime or attempted suicide under care	5.60	.01	.149	.69

References

Abelson, H., and P. Fishburne. 1973. "Drug Experience, Attitudes and Related Behavior Among Adolescents and Adults." In National Commission on Marijuana and Drug Abuse, *Drug Use in America: Problem in Perspective*, Vol. 1. Washington, D.C.: U.S. Government Printing Office, pp. 488-861.

Abelson, H., P. Fishburne, and I. Cisin. 1977. *National Survey on Drug Abuse: 1977, Vol. 1: Main Findings*. Princeton, N.J.: Response Analysis.

Altman, Lawrence. 1986. "Drug Tests Gain Precision, But Can Be Inaccurate." *New York Times*, September 16, p. A-17.

Bale, R. N., W. W. Van Stone, J. M. Kuldau, T. M. Engelsing, R. M. Elashoff, and V. P. Zarcone. 1980. "Therapeutic Communities vs. Methadone Maintenance." *Archives of General Psychiatry* 37 (2): 179-193.

Bell, C., and R. Battjes (eds.). 1985. *Prevention Research: Deterring Drug Abuse Among Children and Adults*. NIDA Research Monograph No. 63. Rockville Md.: National Institute on Drug Abuse.

Bensinger, A., and C. Pilkington. 1983. "An Alternative Method in the Treatment of Alcoholism: The United Technologies Corporation Day Treatment Program." *Journal of Occupational Medicine* 25 (4): 300-303.

Bepko, Claudia. 1985. *The Responsibility Trap: A Blueprint for Treating the Alcoholic Family*. New York: The Free Press.

Beschner, G., and A. S. Friedman. 1985. "Treatment of Adolescent Drug Abusers." *International Journal for Addictions* 20 (6,7): 971-993.

Beschner, G., and A. S. Friedman. 1986. *Teen Drug Abuse*. Lexington, Mass.: Lexington Books.

Biase, D., and Y. Hijazi. 1977. "Daytop's Ambulatory Treatment Units: A Study of the Relationship Between Client Pre-program Profiles and Time in Program." Paper presented at National Drug Abuse Conference, San Francisco, Ca., May 7.

Blakeslee, S. 1987. "Nicotine: Harder to Kick." *The New York Times Magazine*, March 29, pp. 22-23, 49-53.

Botvin, G., and T. Wills. 1985. "Personal and Social Skills Training: Cognitive-Behavioral Approaches to Substance Abuse Prevention." In Bell, C., and R. Battjes (eds.), *Prevention Research: Deterring Drug Abuse Among Children and Adults*. NIDA Research Monograph No. 63. Rockville Md.: National Institute on Drug Abuse, pp. 8-49.

Brinkley, J. 1986. "Drug Law Raises More Than Hope." *New York Times*, November 9, op. ed. page.

Bronfenbrenner, U. 1967. "The Split-Level American Family." *The Saturday Review*, October 7, pp. 60-67.

Bronstein, S. 1987. "Study Shows Sharp Rise in Cocaine Use by Suspects in Crimes." *New York Times*, February 19, p. B-1.

Brook, J. S., I. F. Lukoff, and M. Whiteman. 1977. "Correlates of Adolescent Marijuana Use As Related to Age, Sex and Ethnicity." *Yale Journal of Biological Medicine* 50: 303-390.

Brook, J. S., I. F. Lukoff, and M. Whiteman. 1978. "Family Socialization and Adolescent Personality and Their Association With Adolescent Use of Marijuana." *Journal of Genetic Psychology* 133: 261-271.

Brook, J. S., I. F. Lukoff, and M. Whiteman. 1980. "Initiation into Adolescent Marijuana Use." *Journal of Genetic Psychology* 137: 133-142.

Brown, Stephanie. 1985. *Treating the Alcoholic: A Developmental Model of Recovery.* New York: Wiley.

Brunswick, A., and J. Boyle. 1979. "Patterns of Drug Involvement: Developmental and Secular Influences on Age at Initiation," *Youth and Society* 11 (2): 139-162.

Burt Associates, Inc. 1977. *Drug Treatment in New York City and Washington, D. C.— Followup Studies.* National Institute on Drug Abuse, Washington D. C.: Supt. of Documents, U.S. Government Printing Office.

Carroll, J. 1986. "Secondary Prevention: A Pragmatic Approach to the Problem of Substance Abuse Among Adolescents." In Beschner, G. and A. S. Friedman, *Teen Drug Abuse*, Lexington, Ma.: Lexington Books, pp. 164-184.

Chedekel, M., and N. Patel. 1980. "Large Scale Urinalysis for Drugs of Abuse Using a Multi-Methodology Protocol." Paper presented at the meeting of the American Association of Clinical Chemistry, South Fallsburg, N.Y.

Clayton, R. 1980. "The Delinquency and Drug Use Relationship Among Adolescents, A Critical Review." In D. Lettieri and J. Ludford (eds.), *Drug Abuse and the American Adolescent*. NIDA Research Monograph No. 38. Rockville Md.: National Institute on Drug Abuse.

Cloninger, C. K., Christiansen, T. Reich, and I. Gottesman. 1978. "Implications of Sex Differences in the Prevalences of Antisocial Personality, Alcoholism and Criminality for Family Transmission." *Archives of General Psychiatry* 35: 941-951.

Collier, W. V., and Y. A. Hijazi. 1974. "A Followup Study of Former Residents of a Therapeutic Community." *International Journal of Addictions* 9: 805-826.

Collins, G., E. Watson, and G. Zrimec. 1980. "A Hospital Day Care Program for Alcoholics." *General Hospital Psychiatry* 2: 20-22.

Cowan, A.L. 1989. "Parenthood II: The Nest Won't Stay Empty." *The New York Times*, March 12, pp. 1, 30.

DeLeon, G. 1984. "The Therapeutic Community: Study of Effectiveness." Treatment Research Monograph Series. DHHS Pub. No. (ADM) 84-1286. Rockville, Md: National Institute on Drug Abuse.

DeLeon, G., and S. Schwartz. 1984. "The Therapeutic Community: What are the Retention Rates?" *American Journal of Drug and Alcohol Abuse* 10: 2.

Diocese of Rockville Center. 1986. Bureau of Public Information, reported in telephone communication, Rockville Center, New York, October.

Dohrenwend, B., and B. Dohrenwend. 1969. *Social Status and Psychological Disorder*. New York: Wiley.

Dole, V. P., and H. Joseph. 1978. "Long Term Outcome of Patients Treated With Methadone Maintenance." *Annals of the New York Academy of Sciences* 311: 181.

Dunlap, David. 1982. "1.1 Million Jews Residing in City: A Survey Shows." *New York Times*, May 5, p. B-9.

Falco, M. 1987. "Reagan's Drug Policy: A Bust." *New York Times*, January 13, op. ed. page.

Fox, V., and G. Lowe. 1968. "Day-Hospital Treatment of the Alcoholic Patient," *Quarterly Journal of Studies on Alcohol* 29: 634-641.

Glickman, N., and A. Utada. 1983. "Characteristics of Drug Users in Urban Public High Schools." *Project Report to National Institute on Drug Abuse*. Grant No. H81 DA 01675, Rockville, Md., August.

Goldstein, P., W. Abbott, W. Paige, I. Sobel, and F. Soto. 1977. "Tracking Procedures in Follow-up Studies of Drug Abusers." *American Journal of Drug and Alcohol Abuse* 4(1): 21-30.

Goode, E. 1989. *Drugs In American Society: Third Edition*. New York: Alfred Knopf.

Goodwin, D. 1979. "Alcoholism and Heredity: A Review and Hypothesis." *Archives of General Psychiatry* 36: 57-61.

Goodwin, D. et al. 1977. "Psychopathology in Adopted and Nonadopted Daughters of Alcoholics. *Archives of General Psychiatry* 34: 1005-1009.

Gould, L., and I. Lukoff. 1977. "Selecting A Study Design." In L. Johnston, D. Nurco, and L. Robins (eds.), *Conducting Followup Research on Drug Treatment Programs*. Treatment Program Monograph Series, No. 2. Rockville, Md.: National Institute on Drug Abuse.

Gove, W., M. Geerkin, and M. Hughes. 1979. "Drug Use and Mental Health Among A Representative National Sample of Young Adults. *Social Forces* 58 (21): 572-590.

Halikas, J., and J. Rimmer. 1974. "Predictors of Multiple Drug Use." *Archives of General Psychiatry* 31: 414-418.

Halloran, Richard. 1986. "Survey Finds Sharp Drop in Marijuana Use, in the Military, Pentagon Says." *The New York Times*, January 21, p. A-17.

Hendin, H., A. Pollinger, R. Ulman, and A. Carr. 1981. *Adolescent Marijuana Abusers and Their Families*. NIDA Research Monograph Series No. 40. Washington D.C.: U.S. Government Printing Office.

Hollingshead, A., and F. Redlich. 1958. *Social Class and Mental Illness*. New York: Wiley.

Hubbard, R. et al. 1983. "Treatment Outcome Prospective Study (TOPS): Client Characteristics and Behaviors Before, During and After Treatment." Published in F. Tims and J. Ludford (eds.), 1984, *Drug Abuse Treatment Evaluation: Strategies, Progress and Prospects*. NIDA Research Monograph Series, No. 51. Washington D. C.: U.S. Government Printing Office.

Hubbard, R. et al. 1984. Characteristics, Behaviors And Outcomes for Youths in TOPS Study." Research Triangle Institute, Research Triangle Park, N. C. (report submitted to NIDA, Contract No. 271-79-3611, Rockville, Md.), 1983. Cited in G. Beschner and A. Friedman, 1985, "Treatment of Adolescent Drug Abusers." *International Journal for Addictions* 20 (6,7): 971-993.

Huberty, D. J. 1975. "Treating the Adolescent Drug Abuser: A Family Affair." *Contemporary Drug Problems* 4: 179-194.

Hyman, Merton. 1976. "Alcoholics Fifteen Years Later." *Annals of the New York Academy of Sciences* 273: 613-523.

Jessor, R. 1976. "Predicting Time of Onset of Marijuana Use: A Developmental Study of High School Youth." *Journal of Consulting and Clinical Psychology* 44: 125-134.

Jessor, R., J. Chase, and J. Donovan. 1980. "Psychosocial Correlates of Marijuana Use and Problem Drinking in a National Sample of Adolescents." *American Journal of Public Health* 70 (6): 604-613.

Jessor, R., and S. Jessor. 1977. *Problem Behavior and Psychosocial Development—A Longitudinal Study of Youth*. N.Y.: Academic Press.

Joe, G., and R. Hudiburg. 1978. "Behavioral Correlates of Age at First Marijuana Use." *International Journal of the Addictions* 13: 627-637.

Johnson, B., E. Wish, J. Schmeidler, and D. Huizinga. 1986. *Concentration of Delinquent Offending: The Contribution of Serious Drug Involvement to High Rate Delinquency*. New York: Interdisciplinary Research Center.

Johnston, L.D. 1974. "Drug Use During and After High School: Results of a National Longitudinal Study." *American Journal of Public Health* 64: 29-37.

Johnston, L., P. O'Malley, and J. Bachman. 1988. "Illicit Drug Use, Smoking and Drinking by America's High School Students, College Students, And Young Adults, 1975-1987." National Institute on Drug Abuse, Washington D.C.: U.S. Government Printing Office.

Johnston, L., P. O'Malley, and L. Eveland. 1978. "Drugs and Delinquency—A Search for Causal Connections." In D. B. Kandel (ed.), *Longitudinal Research on Drug Use: Empirical Findings and Methodological Issues*. Washington, D.C.: Hemisphere-Wiley, pp. 132-156.

Kandel, D. 1980. "Drug and Drinking Behavior Among Youth." *Annual Review of Sociology* 6: 235-285.

Kandel, D. 1984. "Marijuana Users in Young Adulthood." *Archives of General Psychiatry* 41: 200-209.

Kandel, D.B., D. Treiman, R. Faust, and E. Single. 1976. "Adolescent Involvement in Illicit Drug Use: A Multiple Classification Analysis." *Social Forces* 55: 438-458.

Kandel, D. B., R. C. Kessler, and R. Z. Margulies. 1978. "Antecedents of Adolescent Initiation Into Stages of Drug Use: A Developmental Analyses." In D. B. Kandel (ed.), *Longitudinal Research on Drug Use: Empirical Findings and Methodological Issues*. New York: Wiley.

Kaufman, Edward. 1972. "A Psychiatrist Views an Addict Self-Help Program." *American Journal of Psychiatry* 128: 7, 846-851.

Kaufman, Irving. 1986. "The Battle Over Drug Testing." *The New York Times Magazine*, October 19, pp. 52-53, 59, 64-65.

Kerr, P. 1986. "Increases in Potency of Marijuana Prompt New Warnings for Youths." *New York Times*, September 25, p. A-1.

Kissin, B., and E. Sang. 1973. "Treatment of Heroin Addiction: Multi-modality Approach." *New York State Journal of Medicine* (May): 1059-1065.

Kleber, Herbert. 1970. "The New Haven Methadone Maintenance Program." *The International Journal of the Addictions*, 5 (3): 449-463.

Kleiman, Mark. 1989. *Marijuana: Costs of Abuse, Costs of Control*. Westport, Conn.: Greenwood Press.

Kleinman, Paula. 1978. "Onset of Addiction: A First Attempt at Prediction." *International Journal of Addictions* 13: 1217-1235.

Kleinman, P., E. Wish, S. Deren, and G. Rainone. 1986. "Multiple Drug Use: A Symptomatic Behavior." *Journal of Psychoactive Drugs* 18 (2): 77-86.

Kleinman, P., E. Wish, S. Deren, G. Rainone, and E. Morehouse. 1987. "Daily Marijuana Use and Problem Behaviors Among Adolescents." *The International Journal of the Addictions* 22.

Kleinman, P., E. Wish, S. Deren, and G. Rainone. 1985. "In Search of the "Pure" Marijuana Client: MARS Working Document #2." Unpublished, Narcotic and Drug Research, Inc., 2 World Trade Center, N.Y.

Kolbert, Elizabeth. 1987. "Youth's Buying of Alcohol Fell in '86." *The New York Times,* February 2, p. B-2.

Kosten, T., B. Rounsaville, and H. Kleber. 1985. "Parental Alcoholism Among Opioid Addicts." *Journal of Nervous and Mental Disease* 173: 461-469.

Kosten, T., B. Rounsaville, and H. Kleber. 1986. "A 2.5 Year Follow-up of Treatment Retention and Re-entry Among Opioid Addicts." *Journal of Substance Abuse Treatment* 3 (3): 181-190.

Lennard, H. et al. 1971. *Mystification and Drug Misuse.* New York: Harper and Row.

Long Island Regional Planning Board. 1982. *Population 1980: Race and Spanish Origin, Data From The 1980 Census of Population and Housing.* Hauppauge, New York (June).

Maddux, J., and David Desmond. 1981. *Careers of Opioid Users.* New York: Praeger.

Maddux, J. F., and L. K. McDonald. 1973. "Status of 100 San Antonio Addicts After Admission to Methadone Maintenance." *Drug Forum* 2: 239.

Mai, L., S. Pedrick, and M. Greene. 1980. "The Learning Laboratory." Treatment Research Monograph. DHHS Publication No. (ADM) 80-928. Rockville, Md: National Institute on Drug Abuse.

McCaul, K., R. Glasgow, H. O'Neil, V. Freeborn, and B. Rump. 1982. "Predicting Adolescent Smoking." *The Journal of School Health* 52 (August): 342-346.

McGoldrick, Monica. 1982. "Irish Families." In M. McGoldrick, J. Pearce, and J. Giordano, *Ethnicity and Family Therapy.* New York: Guilford Press.

McLachlan, J. and R. Stein. 1982. "Evaluation of a Day Clinic for Alcoholics." *Journal of Studies on Alcohol* 43 (3): 261-272.

McLellan, A. T., L. Luborsky, G. Woody, and C. O'Brien, 1980. "An Improved Diagnostic Instrument For Substance Abuse Patients: The Addictions Severity Index." *Journal of Nervous and Mental Disorders* 168: 26-33.

Mellinger, G., R. Somers, and D. Manheimer. 1975. "Drug Use Research Items Pertaining to Personality and Interpersonal Relations: A Working Paper for Research Investigators." In D. Lettieri (ed.), *Predicting Adolescent Drug Abuse: A Review of Issues, Methods and Correlates.* DHEW Pub. No. (ADM) 76-299, National Institute on Drug Abuse, Washington, D.C.: U.S. Government Printing Office.

Mellinger, G. et al. 1978. "Psychic Distress, Life Crisis, and the Use of Psychotherapeutic Medications." *Archives of General Psychiatry* 35: 1045-1052.

Miller, J.D. 1983. *National Survey on Drug Abuse: Main Findings, 1982.* Rockville, Md.: National Institute on Drug Abuse.

Murphy, H. 1975. "Alcoholism and Schizophrenia in the Irish: A Review." *Transcultural Psychiatric Research* 12: 116-139.

Nassau County Planning Commission. 1985. *Nassau County, New York: Date Book*. Mineola, New York.

Nehemkis, A., M. Macari, and D. Lettieri. (eds.) 1976. *Drug Abuse Instrument Handbook*. Research Issues #12, U.S. Dept. of Health and Human Services, DHHS Pub. No. (ADM) 82-394. Rockville, Md.: National Institute on Drug Abuse.

Newcomb, M., and P. Bentler, 1988. *Consequences of Adolescent Drug Use*. Newbury Park, CA.: Sage Publications.

NIDA Capsules, 1986. Rockville Md.: Press Office of the National Institute on Drug Abuse. (November).

Noble, Kenneth. 1986. "Should Employers Be Able to Test For Drug Use?" *The New York Times*, April 17, p. A-25.

Noone, R. J., and R. C. Reddig. 1976. "Case Studies in the Family Treatment of Drug Abuse." *Family Process* 15: 325-332.

Norusis, Marija. 1986. *SPSS/PC+*. Chicago: Ill.: SPSS Inc.

Nye, I., and L. Hoffman, 1963. (eds.) *The Employed Mother in America*. Chicago: Rand McNally.

Parry, H. I., Cisin, M. Balter, G. Mellinger, and D. Manheimer. 1974. "Increased Alcohol Intake As A Coping Mechanism for Psychic Distress." In R. Cooperstock (ed.) *Social Aspects of the Medical Use of Psychotropic Drugs*. Ontario: Addiction Research Foundation.

Paton, S. R., Kessler, and D. Kandel. 1977. "Depressive Mood and Illegal Drug Use: A Longitudinal Analysis." *Journal of Genetic Psychology* 131: 267-289.

Pederson, L. and N. Lefcoe. 1985. "Cross-Sectional Analysis of Variables Related to Cigarette Smoking in Late Adolescence." *Journal of Drug Education* 15 (3): 225-240.

Pin, E. J., J. M. Martin, and J. F. Walsh. 1976. "A Followup Study of 300 Ex-clients of a Drug Free Narcotic Treatment Program in New York City." *American Journal of Drug and Alcohol Abuse* 3: 397-407.

Rabkin, J. and E. Streuning. 1976. "Ethnicity, Social Class and Mental Illness in New York City: A Social Area Analysis of Five Ethnic Groups." Working Paper No. 17. New York: Institute on Pluralism and Group Identity.

Radosevich, Marcia, L. Lanza-Kaduce, R. Akers, and M. Krohn. 1979. "The Sociology of Adolescent Drug and Drinking Behavior, A Review of the State of The Field, Part 1." *Deviant Behavior* 1: 15-35.

Reilly, D. M. 1975. "Family Factors in the Etiology and Treatment of Youthful Drug Abuse." *Family Therapy* 2: 149-171.

Reinhold, R. 1982. "An 'Overwhelming' Violence-TV Tie." *New York Times*, May 6, p. C-27.

Richards, L. 1986."Perspectives on Drug Use in the United States." *Drugs and Society* 1 (1): 111-126.

Riche, M. F. 1987. "Mysterious Young Adults." *American Demographics* 9 (2): 38-43.

Roberts, B., and J. Myers. 1954. "Religion, National Origin, Immigration and Mental Illness." *American Journal of Psychiatry* 110: 759-764.

Robins, L., D. H. Davis, and E. Wish. 1977. "Detecting Predictors of Rare Events: Demographic, Family and Personal Deviance as Predictors in Stages in the Progression Toward Narcotic Addiction." In J. S. Straus, B. Haroutun, and M. Roff (eds.), *The Origins and Course of Psychopathology*. N.Y.: Plenum, pp. 379-406.

Rush, T. V. 1979. "Predicting Treatment Outcomes for Juvenile and Young Adult Clients in the Pennsylvania Substance-Abuse System." In G. M. Beschner and A. S. Friedman (eds.), *Youth Drug Abuse: Problems, Issues and Treatment*. Lexington, Mass.: D.C. Heath.

Russe, B., D. McBride, C. McCoy, and J. Inciardi. 1977. "An Analysis of the Accessibility and Nonaccessibility of Patients in a Followup Study." *The International Journal of the Addictions* 12 (6): 707-716.

Sanua, V. 1960. "Sociocultural Factors in Responses to Stressful Life Situations: The Behavior of Aged Amputees As An Example." *Journal of Health and Human Behavior* 1: 17-24.

Schnaiberg, A., and S. Goldenberg, 1989. "From Empty Nest to Crowded Nest: The Dynamics of Incompletely-Launched Young Adults." *Social Problems* 36 (3): 251-269.

Sells, S.B., and D. D. Simpson. 1974. *Effectiveness of Drug Abuse Treatments, Vol. 1, Evaluation of Treatments*. Cambridge, Mass.: Ballinger.

Sells, S. B., and D. D. Simpson. 1979. "Evaluation of Treatment Outcomes for Youths in the Drug Abuse Reporting Program (DARP): A Followup Study." In G. M. Beschner and A. S. Friedman (eds.), *Youth Drug Abuse: Problems, Issues and Treatment*. Lexington, Mass.: D. C. Heath.

Simpson, D. D. 1979. "The Relation of Time Spent in Drug Abuse Treatment to Posttreatment Outcome." *American Journal of Psychiatry* 136 (11): 1449-1453.

Simpson, D. D., L. J. Savage, and S. B. Sells, 1978. *Date Book on Drug Treatment Outcomes: Followup Study of 1969-72 Admissions to the DARP*. (Report 78-IV). Fort Worth, Tx.: Texas Christian Univ., Institute of Behavioral Research.

Simpson, D. D., and S. B. Sells. 1982. "Effectiveness of Treatment for Drug Abuse: An Overview of the DARP Research Program." *Advances in Alcohol and Substance Abuse* 2 (1): 7-29.

Simpson, D. D., G. W. Joe, W. E. Lehman, and S. B. Sells. 1986. "Addiction Careers: Etiology, Treatment and 12-Year Follow-up Outcomes." *Journal of Drug Issues* 16 (1): 107-122.

Smith, G., and C. Fogg. 1975. "Teenage Drug Use: A Search for Causes and Consequences." In D. Lettieri (ed.), *Predicting Adolescent Drug Abuse: A Review of Issues, Methods and Correlates*. DHEW Pub. No. (ADM) 76-299, National Institute of Drug Abuse, Washington D.C.: U.S. Government Printing Office.

Srole, Leo, T. Langner, S. Michael, M. Opler, and T. Rennie. 1962. *Mental Health in the Metropolis: Midtown Manhattan Study*. Vol 1. New York: McGraw Hill.

Stanton, M. D., T. Todd, D. Heard, S. Kirshner, J. Kleiman, D. Mowatt, P. Riley, S. Scott, and J. Van Deusen. 1978. "Heroin Addiction as a Family Phenomenon: A New Conceptual Model." *American Journal of Drug and Alcohol Abuse* 5: 125-150.

Stimmel, B. et al. 1978. "Detoxification for Methadone Maintenance: Risk Factors Associated With Relapse to Narcotic Use." *Annals of the New York Academy of Sciences* 311: 173-180.

Tims, F. 1981. "Treatment Research Report: Effectiveness of Drug Abuse Treatment Programs." DHHS Pub. No. (ADM) 81-1143. Rockville, Md.: National Institute on Drug Abuse.

Tricarico, Donald. 1984. *The Italians of Greenwich Village: The Social Structure and Transformation of an Ethnic Community*. Staten Island, N.Y.: Center for Migration Studies of N.Y.

U.S. Department of Health Education and Welfare, 1970. "Changes in Smoking Habits Between 1955 and 1966." Washington, D.C.: Government Printing Office.

U.S. Department of Health Education and Welfare. 1977. "The Smoking Digest: Progress Report on a Nation Kicking the Habit." Washington, D.C.: Government Printing Office.

Vaillant, G. 1978. "A 20-year Followup of New York Narcotic Addicts." *Archives of General Psychiatry* 29: 237-241.

Weil, A. 1972. *The Natural Mind: A New Way of Looking at Drugs and the Higher Consciousness.* Boston: Houghton Mifflin.

Wilentz, A. 1987. "Teen Suicide," *Time Magazine*, March 23, pp. 12-13.

Winn, J. 1981. "A Cultural Enrichment Program for Youth." Treatment Research Notes. Rockville, Md.: National Institute on Drug Abuse.

Wish, E., B. Johnson, D. Strug, M. Chedekel, and D. Lipton. 1983. "Are Urine Tests Good Indicators of the Validity of Self-Reports of Drug Use? It Depends on the Test." Unpublished report of the Interdisciplinary Research Center, Narcotic and Drug Research, Inc. 2 World Trade Center, New York, N.Y. (June).

Zborowski, M. 1969. *People in Pain.* San Francisco: Jossey-Bass.

Zola, I. 1966. "Culture and Symptoms: An Analysis of Patients' Presenting Complaints." *American Sociological Review* 5: 141-155.

Index

About the Author

WILLIAM FEIGELMAN is Professor and Chair of the Sociology Department at Nassau Community College, Garden City, New York, where he has taught for the last twenty-four years. He is co-author of *Chosen Children* (Praeger, 1983).